The Complete Book of
Oriental Yoga
Hatha and Taoist Yoga for the Seasons

By Michael Hetherington
(L. Ac, Yoga Teacher)

Copyright 2014 Michael Hetherington

By law, this work is protected by copyright. Therefore, no one is permitted to copy, broadcast, transmit, show or play in public, adapt or change in any way the content of this book - for any other purpose whatsoever - without prior written permission from Michael Hetherington.

www.michaelhetherington.com.au

info@michaelhetherington.com.au

Australia

Disclaimer
All material in this book is provided for your information only and may not be construed as medical advice or instruction. No action or inaction should be taken based solely on the contents of this information; instead, readers should consult the appropriate health professionals on any matter relating to their health and well-being.

The information and opinions expressed here are believed to be accurate, based on the best judgment available to the authors, and readers who fail to consult with the appropriate health authorities assume the risk of any injuries. The publisher is not responsible for errors or omissions.

Acknowledgements

I would like to thank the yoga teachers at Zen Central in Brisbane, Australia who first introduced me to a fusion of Indian yoga and Oriental medicine. They also taught me how yoga can be practiced in a fun and joyful way. I would like to thank my partner, Angela Hammond, for the help with photos, the graphic design and ongoing support. I would also like to thank the yoga community in Australia and around the world who continue to inspire and motivate me. And of course, I would like to offer a special thanks to all the saints, sages and mystics of the past who dedicated their lives to the path of truth.

About the Author

Michael Hetherington is a qualified acupuncturist, health practitioner and yoga teacher based in Brisbane, Australia. He has a keen interest in mind-body medicine, energetic anatomy, yoga nidra and Buddhist style meditation. Inspired by the teachings of many, he has learnt that a light-hearted, joyful approach to life serves best.

www.michaelhetherington.com.au

Other Titles by Author:

Chakra Balancing Made Simple and Easy

How to Do Restorative Yoga

The Little Book of Yin

Meditation Made Simple

How to Learn Acupuncture

EFT Through the Chakras

Oriental Yoga

Table of Contents

INTRODUCTION 9
YOGA AND THE SEASONS 11

PART 1 - ORIENTAL YOGA FUNDAMENTALS 13
INTRODUCTION TO THE 5-ELEMENTS/PHASES 14
YIN AND YANG AND THE WHOLE SHI-BANG! 18
MERIDIANS AND CHAKRAS 21
INTRODUCTION TO ORIENTAL DIET THERAPY 23
MUSCLES ASSOCIATED WITH THE ORGANS 28
PRINCIPLES OF ORIENTAL YOGA 29
FUNDAMENTALS OF A YOGA CLASS 33

PART 2 - YOGA FOR THE SEASONS 43
EARTH ELEMENT 44
EARTH ORGAN PHYSIOLOGY 47
THE EARTH ELEMENT MERIDIANS 52
MUSCLES ASSOCIATED WITH THE STOMACH 55
MUSCLES ASSOCIATED WITH THE SPLEEN 57
ASANAS (POSTURES) FOR LATE SUMMER 60
EARTH ELEMENT DAILY LIFESTYLE PRACTICES 71
SUPPORTING THE OTHER ELEMENTS TO ASSIST THE EARTH ELEMENT 73
FOOD / ORIENTAL DIET THERAPY ~ LATE SUMMER 74

HERBS TO SUPPORT THE STOMACH AND SPLEEN 76
LATE SUMMER MEDITATIONS 77

METAL ELEMENT 79
METAL ORGAN PHYSIOLOGY 81
THE METAL ELEMENT MERIDIANS 84
MUSCLES ASSOCIATED WITH THE LUNGS 86
MUSCLES ASSOCIATED WITH THE LARGE INTESTINE 89
ASANAS (POSTURES) FOR AUTUMN 92
METAL ELEMENT DAILY LIFESTYLE PRACTICES...................... 106
SUPPORTING THE OTHER ELEMENTS TO ASSIST THE METAL ELEMENT 107
FOOD / ORIENTAL DIET THERAPY ~ AUTUMN 108
HERBS TO SUPPORT LUNGS AND LARGE INTESTINE 110
AUTUMN MEDITATIONS 112

WATER ELEMENT 116
WATER ORGAN PHYSIOLOGY 119
THE WATER ELEMENT MERIDIANS 122
MUSCLES ASSOCIATED WITH THE KIDNEYS........................... 125
MUSCLES ASSOCIATED WITH THE BLADDER 129
ASANAS (POSTURES) FOR WINTER 132
WATER ELEMENT DAILY LIFESTYLE PRACTICES...................... 145
SUPPORTING THE OTHER ELEMENTS TO ASSIST THE WATER ELEMENT 147
FOOD / ORIENTAL DIET THERAPY ~ WINTER 149
HERBS TO SUPPORT THE KIDNEYS AND BLADDER 151

Oriental Yoga

WINTER MEDITATIONS 152

WOOD ELEMENT 154
WOOD ORGAN PHYSIOLOGY 157
THE WOOD ELEMENT MERIDIANS 160
MUSCLES ASSOCIATED WITH THE LIVER 163
MUSCLES ASSOCIATED WITH THE GALLBLADDER 165
ASANAS (POSTURES) FOR SPRING 166
WOOD ELEMENT DAILY LIFESTYLE PRACTICES 179
SUPPORTING THE OTHER ELEMENTS TO ASSIST THE WOOD ELEMENT 181
FOOD / ORIENTAL DIET THERAPY ~ SPRING 182
HERBS TO SUPPORT THE LIVER AND GALLBLADDER 184
SPRING MEDITATIONS 185

FIRE ELEMENT 188
FIRE ORGAN PHYSIOLOGY 191
THE FIRE ELEMENT MERIDIANS 194
MUSCLES ASSOCIATED WITH THE HEART 196
MUSCLES ASSOCIATED WITH THE SMALL INTESTINE 197
ASANAS (POSTURES) FOR SUMMER 199
FIRE ELEMENT DAILY LIFESTYLE PRACTICES 215
SUPPORTING THE OTHER ELEMENTS TO ASSIST THE FIRE ELEMENT 217
FOOD / ORIENTAL DIET THERAPY ~ SUMMER 218
HERBS TO SUPPORT THE HEART AND SMALL INTESTINE 220
SUMMER MEDITATIONS 221

CONCLUSION 224
RECOMMENDED READING 225
RESOURCES 226

Introduction

"Those who flow as life flows, know they need no other force"
~ Lao Tzu

    Oriental Yoga is a fusion of traditional Indian Hatha yoga with traditional Oriental medicine and Taoist cosmology. The aim of applying this knowledge is, like all yoga's and spiritual paths, to help the practitioner align with the natural cosmic forces of the universe. When one aligns with these natural forces, the path becomes more harmonious, more easeful and more joyful, for these are the innate qualities of the universal way.

This book aims to give the yoga practitioner an understanding of basic Taoist philosophical concepts, as well as provide practical tools and techniques to apply this theory to enhance one's daily life. As do all systems and philosophies, they are not absolute, as the absolute lies beyond the world of concepts and ideals. Therefore, this philosophical framework serves more as a practice to prepare one to springboard toward the absolute.

The aim of this book is to help one come to a deeper understanding of the natural forces at play and how we fit into this dance we call life. I hope to equip you with tools and techniques to assist you in making useful and beneficial lifestyle adjustments and also influence your yoga practice so that it may be in harmony with the natural order of things. I also hope to encourage and inspire a willing attitude, so that you remain open and allow intuition and flow to become an everyday reality and occurrence. When we find this flow in our daily lives, joy and happiness are not far away. In truth, they are already there. When we cultivate this flow in our daily lives, the mind becomes steadier and intuition—our inner wisdom beyond the world of thoughts—becomes a lot stronger and more prevalent in our lives, saving us a great deal of stress and exertion.

The first part of this book aims to cover the fundamental principles and overarching philosophical approach to the practices of Oriental yoga. The second part of the book is focused more on practical aspects, which take into consideration the 5 elements and the 5 seasons.

I have found this information to be very helpful and useful in my life, as well as in the lives of those who are familiar with it. Therefore, I'm sure it will serve you in many beneficial ways, also.

Thank you for taking the time to pick up this book. I'm positive it will help you make a stronger connection with the natural forces of life and also help with the deepening of your yoga practice.

Yoga and the Seasons

There is no doubt that energy moves through us differently according to the time of day, the climatic conditions, the attitudes we harbor and the cycles of the moon, just to name a few. With the natural flow of seasons, so too it makes sense that our yoga practice is to reflect these changes.

Throughout Chinese medicine and Taoist thought, the aim is to find and establish harmony by aligning with the natural flow of life. To live the path of least resistance means that one is aligned with nature and with the divine expression of life itself. These ideas are not limited to Chinese thought and can be found throughout ayurvedic medicine (said to be the oldest medicine on the planet), yogic science and many other traditions and cultures who place great importance on learning from the changes in nature.

No amount of individualized effort, willpower or force can be sustained and supported when working against the natural flow of nature and the universe. Only when one comes to flow with the natural forces of life and the universe, can one begin to uncover the deep peace, joy and stillness that reside within.

In the western world, we are familiar with the four seasons - spring, summer, autumn and winter. However, in the Taoist understanding of time and change they devised five seasons. They are spring, summer, late summer, autumn and winter. The extra season is called late summer and refers to the end of the summer season when it becomes more humid. In section 2 of this book we will explore each of the 5 elements in much greater detail.

Oriental Yoga Fundamentals

Part 1

"Nature does not hurry, yet everything is accomplished."

~ Lao Tzu

Introduction to the 5-Elements/Phases

Within Traditional Chinese Medicine and Taoist cosmology, the 5 element theory was most likely conceived around 476 - 221 BC. This was really one of the first developments of science, as they came to realize that natural phenomena was actually produced and created through the interacting relationships of natural elements and were not, therefore, the acts of Gods or unseen beings that reigned havoc on the earth when they were not pleased or showered gifts from above when they were happy.

This was a revolutionary breakthrough in the way they viewed life and the process of disease. Over time—mainly through their observations—they focused on five primary elements and their inter-relationships within all physical phenomena. They also drew connections between these elements and the mental, emotional and spiritual dimensions of the human being. This theory did not die out through time. Instead, it became even more solidified into the theory and practice of traditional Chinese medicine and Taoism to this day; therefore, making it one of the oldest and most field-tested theories and medicines on the planet.

Let's have a closer look at these 5 elements:

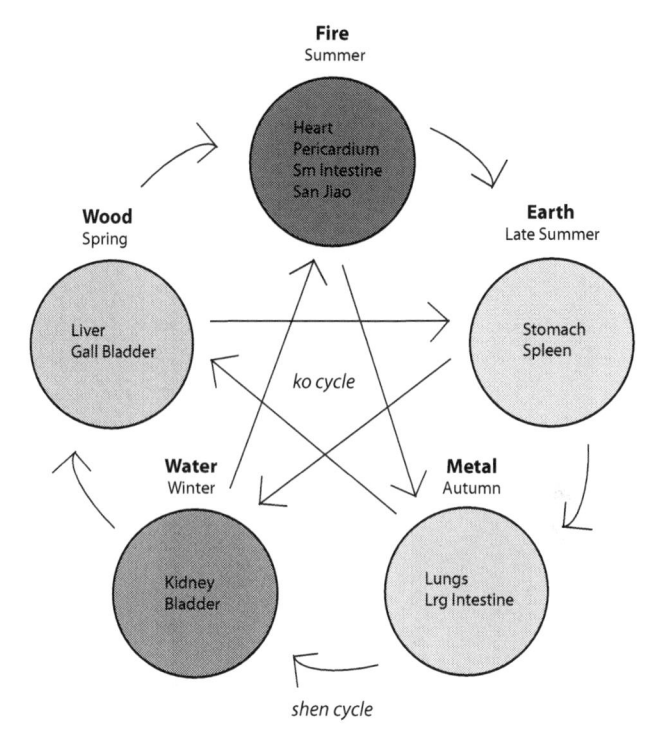

Figure 1.1

The 5-Elements are:

Earth – Late Summer - Stomach and Spleen
Metal – Autumn - Large Intestine and Lungs
Water – Winter - Kidney and Bladder
Wood – Spring - Liver and Gallbladder
Fire – Summer - Heart, Small Intestine, Pericardium and San Jiao (temperature regulator)

As illustrated above in figure 1.1, there are two different types of relationships at play. One is called the *Shen* (nurturing) cycle and the other is the *Ko* (controlling) cycle.

Shen (nurturing) Cycle Explained

The *Shen* is described as the generating or nurturing cycle, likened to that of the relationship between a mother and her son. The energy flows from one element to the other in a cyclic fashion. Problems arise when the energy becomes stuck, stagnant, or weak in a particular element, therefore affecting the following element. For example, if the Fire element becomes stagnant, blocked; or the fire simply gets put out or dampened, it causes problems for the Earth element. Then we will get signs and symptoms of disease within the Earth element, and in the case of treatment, we will need to treat the Fire element alongside the Earth element so the *Shen* cycle can be re-established.

The *Ko* (controlling) Cycle Explained

The *Ko* cycle is also described as the controlling cycle because it is likened to that of the relationship between a grandmother and a grandson; well, in traditional families anyway. The grandmother has a strong influence on the grandson's life and choices. So if we use the same ideas as in the *Shen* example, where the Earth element has become weak and we have signs and symptoms of the Earth element' problems, it could well be due to the Wood element controlling Earth. Wood can easily overpower the Earth element, as the liver tends to get hot and irritated easily. Or, the Wood element may simply be acting to cut the Earth element off by not giving it any energy and both of these examples would leave the Earth element in all sorts of problems. Therefore, sometimes we need to treat the Wood element to treat the Earth element and so on.

It's not necessary to fully grasp these concepts; yet, they prove very helpful when treating any illness or any signs and symptoms of imbalance. If we become familiar with the inter-relationships between the elements, we can really work out where the initial problem may have arisen and therefore, treat the underlying _cause_ and not just the _symptoms,_ as is what happens in most cases.

Yin and Yang and the Whole Shi-Bang!

What about yin and yang? Where does this fit into it? Yin and yang are said to be the first expression of energy from the primordial ONE or *Wuji* as it is referred to in Chinese. The energy that shone forth from the primordial ONE was an energetic force known as Qi (a highly intelligent, electrical fabric also sometimes referred to as bioenergy). In order for it to come into existence, it separated itself from the ONE and therefore, divided itself into duality – known as yin and yang. We humans have called it yin and yang and to us it appears to be a divided force, but this is not entirely true. It is not actually divided at all, but rather, just an expression of the ONE source. For humans to talk about it and conceptualize it, we need to divide it into yin and yang. Yin and yang is the world of duality, of light and dark, of sun and moon, of right and wrong, of language, of division and of mental conceptualization. From the yin and yang division, this Qi force then continues to divide and split further into the 5 elements to create the world of matter. Man's body is made from the 5 elements, his mind is made up of primarily thought, which is dualistic in nature (yin and yang), and his spirit or heart is connected to the ONE or the *Wuji*, yet many humans are not aware of this.

One of man's biggest hindrances to self-realization is his over-identification with the intellect and the yin and yang of things. It is, of course, helpful to a degree to harness and understand the yin and yang of our world and our intellect. However, man has little faith or experience in cultivating and nurturing the relationship with the source that resides in the heart, and this sense of disconnection reduces one's capacity to live fully. All enlightened beings sit firmly in the source, the field beyond yin and yang, beyond the limitation of mind. As long as one has a physical body, the body will always be influenced by the 5 elements, yet his or her heart can be free.

When man aligns his body, mind and heart with the universal flow of this expression of energy, this is called the Tao or the Way of the spiritual warrior. Figure 1.2 is an illustration to help express this cosmology.

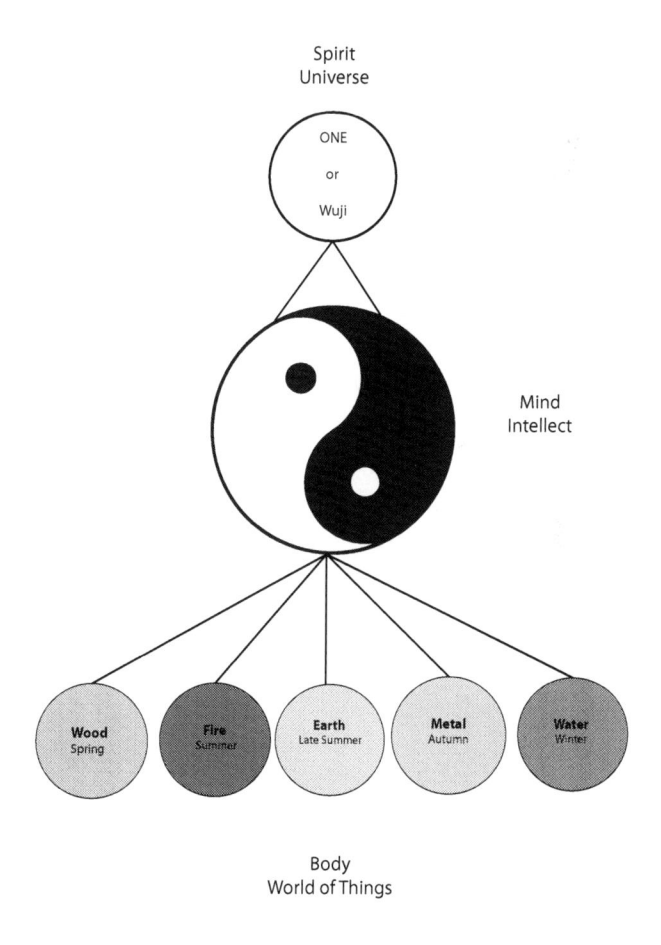

Figure 1.2

The Oriental Yoga system is designed to balance the 5 elements, purify the mind and open the heart. We utilize asana (bodily postures), diet and lifestyle to harmonize the physical laws of the 5 elements. We use meditative techniques and contemplative exercises to harmonize and purify the yin and yang of the mind. After some time, when the worlds of mind and matter are purified and harmonized, the door to the heart will open to the true ONE of the universe. The process involves the continual purification and cultivation of mind and matter harmonization so that this doorway becomes wider and the path to the heart becomes more established. Eventually, as one gets fully established on the path of the heart, at some point, the influence of the 5 elements and the intellectualizing mind will fall away in its significance. But first, focus on harmonizing the 5 elements and working at calming and purifying the mind. The rest will reveal itself when the practitioner is ready.

Meridians and Chakras

As we move into the field of "energetic anatomy" we begin to uncover the Chakra system and the meridian system. The Chakras, which are known more commonly in the traditional Indian yogic systems, are referred to as major energy centers, wheels, or vortexes where immense amounts of Qi energy is processed and generated. There are 7 primary chakras that are located along the length of human spine. The Chakras process and then distribute great amounts of Qi out to the rest of the body via the meridian channels or *"nadi"* channels as they are called in the Yoga's. In this way, both the Chakras and the meridian pathways are intrinsically connected and therefore during any treatment process, both energetic systems will need to be taken into consideration. The Chakras are subtle, so much as to say that most humans cannot see them using their physical eyes, however most humans can feel and sense them both consciously and unconsciously. The Chakras are very powerful and have the capacity to influence all levels of a human being from the physical, through to the mental, emotional levels as well as the spiritual.

The meridians are a vast network of energy channels that distribute the Qi and move blood around the body. They can be likened to that of a complex river and irrigation system that distributes nourishment and life giving water throughout the land. When the meridian system or Chakra system are impaired in any way, it can give rise to any number of physical, mental or spiritual imbalances. The traditional Chinese Taoists mainly focused on, and mapped out in great detail, 14 main channel pathways that are used in traditional Chinese medicine today. In the pictures used in this book, and in most Oriental medical literature, we mainly focus on the meridian pathways where they come to the surface of the body. It's important to know that these meridians also run their networks deep within the body. The reason we primarily focus on the channels that come to the surface of the body is because they are more accessible to us and therefore easier to treat. To access the deeper networks of these meridians, especially in the case of certain illnesses that become very established and internalized, herbal medicines, herbal tinctures, diet and meditational practices are recommended, as they have better access to the internal environment.

Each organ has its own meridian network that acts to nourish, feed and express it. Three of these meridians aren't directly related to an organ and therefore play an energetic role only. The meridians for the organs are lungs, large intestine, kidney, bladder, liver, gallbladder, heart, pericardium, small intestine, stomach and spleen. The three extra meridians that aren't associated with an organ are Ren (central), Du (back) and the San Jiao (temperature regulator).

For the study and practice of Oriental Yoga, we mainly work with the 14 main meridians and to a lesser extent, 3 of the primary chakras. The 3 Chakras being the 2nd Chakra (*Hara* as it is known in Japanese and *dan tien* as it is known in Chinese) the 4th Chakra, more commonly known as the heart Chakra (*Shen* in Chinese medicine) and the 6th Chakra known more commonly as the third eye.

Introduction to Oriental Diet Therapy

In Oriental diet therapy, the approach to food is quite different than the common approaches in the western world. One of the principles, especially if one is unwell or weak, is to only eat well-cooked foods – foods in the form of soups, stews, casseroles and porridges and drink only warm tea and warm water. If we put in foods that are already broken down and warm, then the body can absorb it quickly and efficiently without requiring a great deal of internal energy to process it.

It is believed that each food or herb has either warming or cooling properties and depending on the person, season and/or illness, we adjust the foods and herbs to reflect the required internal warming or cooling for balancing the system. In relation to the seasons, because summer and spring have a lot of heat in the atmosphere which is also transferred into our bodies, we can get away with eating cooler foods like salads, fruits and raw foods. But in winter and autumn, it is generally recommended to eat more cooked and warm foods to nourish and warm the body. Therefore, it is best to avoid ice cold drinks, ice water and things like ice cream, especially in cooler climates or when sick or unwell.

For the traditional yogi and spiritual aspirant, a vegetarian diet is often encouraged as a way of reducing harm to animals and other living beings. While a vegetarian diet is recommended for the serious yogi, obtaining the right nutrients from a vegetarian diet is quite a science and therefore a yogi who practices vegetarianism will often also need to become somewhat of a nutritionist. To go into a vegetarian diet without adequate education in nutrition can lead the student into all kinds of unnecessary health problems, which will actually distract and hinder the practice of yoga.

For example, in order to follow a path into vegetarianism, one must become familiar with the amino acids found in proteins. Proteins are the fundamental building blocks of human tissue and therefore essential for the growth and maintenance of a healthy human body. Proteins can be found in vegetable matter, but those in vegetable matter are considered "incomplete" because they only carry a limited number of the necessary amino acids. Therefore, when eating only vegetable matter, one must consume two complementary sources of incomplete proteins in order to make up a "complete" protein, which is most beneficial to the body. Meat is considered "complete" because it carries a majority of the necessary amino acids and therefore there is no matching of other foods required.

In Oriental medicine, meat is recommended for most body types and is considered a necessary component for those who are young and growing, or for those who are ill or weak. Taking meat in excess is potentially just as detrimental as not eating enough meat and therefore the rule of balance and common sense applies here too. Meat is seen as a necessary ingredient to keep blood and Qi strong and abundant. Eating meat does not always indicate that one is causing harm to another being. Through the practices of gratitude and mindful eating, negative karmas from eating meat can be effectively dissolved. In Oriental medicine it is said that there are only a few, rare people who can handle a raw, vegetarian food diet. A person gifted with a good constitution, a well-defined and strong body and fiery digestion is a sign of such a person. Though for most of us, taking on only a diet of raw and vegetarian foods without thorough education in nutrition and a suitable body type can cause unnecessary disturbance and deficiency in our Qi and blood stores.

Fasting is a recommended practice to undergo at least once a year. The primary purpose of a fast is not so much about detoxing the body, but about detoxing the mind. The act of fasting trains the mind to overcome attachments to those things associated with pleasure; food being the primary one. Therefore, the person who fasts works to cultivate a strong resolve which often proves beneficial to many other aspects of the yogi's life.

The quality and regularity of your bowel movements provide an accurate indicator of your internal organs' health. It's important to spend a little time explaining what an ideal bowel motion involves because it is rarely discussed. Generally speaking, a bowel motion at least once a day is a good indicator and to have the bowel motion before breakfast is considered the ideal time to do it. The ideal bowel motion is brown in color, not too dry, meaning not pebble like, and not too wet and loose. Having a bowel motion should be rather quick, come without much effort and without the need to wipe much afterwards. It should also not produce a smell that peels the paint off the walls. If you consistently have signs of unhealthy bowel motions, then it would be advised to seek out a health practitioner to help steer your digestive system back on track. An acupuncturist, herbalist, naturopath or general medicine practitioner will all be able to offer you some assistance. It may be a little embarrassing to talk about this to your health practitioner but it is very important to address it early on because it can easily lead to further health problems later on.

Constipation is a regular occurrence in the modernized lifestyle and is a sure indication of an imbalance. Usually, it stems from energy stagnation and can often be cleared by more physical movement, a reduction in breads, pastas and other heavy types of foods and by adding some digestive tonics and stimulants to the digestive system such as some chili, lemon water or apple cider vinegar. Emotionally, constipation is connected to being unable to "let go" and this can manifest as constipation. In the Metal Element chapter found later in this book, we address this issue in much more detail. If you are unable to correct the constipation through your own efforts it's advised to seek out assistance from a health practitioner.

General Principles of Oriental Diet Therapy:

- Eat to only 70-80% full. Overeating taxes life force and damages the stomach and spleen organs. It is also good for mental training. Overeating is a sign of attachment to the senses and a loss of equanimity of the mind.

- Eat with mindfulness, patience, with minimal distractions and chew thoroughly.

- Avoid extreme temperatures of foods. This means to avoid ice cold drinks such as ice water and avoid foods like ice cream. It is also better to avoid overly spiced foods, foods cooked on open flames and foods that are dried out.

- In most cases and especially in any case of illness, weakness, age or poor digestion, it is recommended to eat well cooked foods such as soups, stews, congees and casseroles. Only those with a strong constitution can handle raw foods for extended periods.

- Vegetarianism is recommended for the serious yogi, however education in nutrition is a must to avoid energetic and blood deficiencies.

- Meat in most cases is recommended, especially for the young and for those who are ill or weak.

- The quality and regularity of your bowel motions provide an accurate indicator of your internal organ health. It's important to address any consistent signs of constipation or ongoing wet or loose stools. You can do this through adjusting diet, adding digestive tonics and adding more dynamic physical movements. If these options don't prove helpful, seek assistance form a health practitioner.

Muscles Associated with the Organs

Thanks to the good work of chiropractic Doctor, George Goodheart, we discovered in the '60s and '70s that each meridian in the Chinese medicine energetic system has a direct relationship with various muscles and neural pathways of the body. This means that, if a meridian was 'out' or not flowing properly, the muscle associated with it would also not be functioning properly; the neuromuscular activity would be somewhat impaired. Therefore, it was found that if you corrected the meridian, the muscle would return to its full function and, similarly, if you corrected the muscle function, the meridian would correct. This was quite an amazing discovery that has essentially added a new dimension to the treatment of energetic dysfunction and the understanding of disease within the body.

Once we know the muscles associated with the meridians and the location of the meridians themselves, we can then apply the appropriate asanas (postures), or indeed any form of movement training that targets these areas of the body to re-establish the correct energetic flow through our systems. The recommended yoga asanas are explored for each meridian in further chapters.

Principles of Oriental Yoga

As with every system of yoga, there are certain principles of the yoga practice that are emphasized more so than others. This is not intended to exclude other yogic practices, but rather, it aims to simply bring focus to certain aspects of the overall yogic practice.

Change is Constant
(Thoughts, Emotions, Experiences, Seasons etc.)

The yogi practices non-attachment to the world of form because the yogi understands change to be a constant phenomenon. The yogi appreciates form as it arises but understands its true nature and therefore allows its passing to occur without resistance. Eventually the yogi will come to a point where they will ask, what is it that does not change?

Trust in the Flow of Life

The universe is infinitely organized and is playing out its process of consciousness evolution, of which we have the privilege to perceive and be a witness to. When we cease trying to control the world or change it to how we think it should be, we come to a place of acceptance and faith in the way things are. When there is trust in this process, we can relax into life and the present moment. Our perception is also altered and the penetration of the smallness is transcended so that one can see all of life unfolding as it is without the need to project wrongness or rightness onto it.

Joy as an Underlying State (Under Emotions)

Joy is an innate, default quality of existence itself and is present beneath all the emotional layers of the human condition. It is subtle yet powerful and is essentially non-form in nature. When all of the various forms and emotions are penetrated through purification of mind and through true seeing, joy is revealed.

Hara is the Physical Centre, the Heart is the Emotional Centre and the Third Eye is the Spiritual Centre of the Human Being

The point just below the belly button, known as the *Hara* in Japanese, and the *Dan Tien* in Chinese, is the centre of the physical aspects of the human being. The Heart centre is the centre of the emotional and mental aspects of the human being and the third eye is the centre of the spiritual body. The yogi cultivates presence, awareness and space within these 3 main areas, with the *Hara* being the foundation that provides grounding for the other aspects to be cultivated.

Become the Witness

The yogi is able to move into the perceptional position of a witness to all sensory experiences, which include the activity of the mind, and therefore is not ruled by them. The yogi investigates the one who is witnessing the senses and when established in this practice, eventually merges with the one who is witnessing all phenomenon.

Cause No Harm

Not only does causing no harm work to support life force in all beings, it helps to eliminate bad karma and support positive karma. Over time, it becomes obvious to the spiritual aspirant that causing no intentional harm is actually a natural state of being and therefore one adjusts to this behavior out of personal and universal choice, not out of obligation or fear.

Karma is caused by the reactionary tendencies towards feelings and sensations as they arise. When these reactions continue to be fuelled and re-affirmed, one continues to re-energize and create similar outcomes and continues the generation of karma. When one comes to a place of non-reactivity and insight regarding feelings and sensations, karma is naturally burned up and eventually extinguished, leaving the yogi free of all karmic affects.

Acceptance of Both Positivity and Negativity

Negativity in its various forms, is a natural part of the human condition and learning to accept, observe and discontinue to feed negativity becomes a yogic practice. In this way negative states are not seen as a failure or something to be ashamed or guilty of, rather negativity is an energy that can be utilized for one's growth and transformation. Both positive and negative states are therefore utilized for burning up past karmas and utilized for self-realization.

Courage and Willingness are Primary Qualities

The yogi understands that one plays the primary role in one's perception of reality and therefore takes responsibility for its outcomes. Courage is necessary to face oneself and willingness is required to continue to place one's attention on purifying one's mind and becoming established in reality.

The Continuous Act of Surrender and Letting Go

We can only be fully alive when we are present and grounded in the present moment. If we continue to place our attention in the past or project our energy into an uncertain future we lose touch with the reality of now. The key to maintaining presence in reality is the continual surrender of what arises without adding further commentary to it. In this way we are able to surrender our feelings, thoughts and sensations as they arise and therefore remain fully in the present moment.

Existence is Enough to Love and be Loved

Unconditional love comes through surrendering the need to have a list of reasons in order to love someone or something. Ones very own existence is seen as a gift of God and this makes it easy to love others and oneself when one comes to understand that to exist is enough.

Fundamentals of a Yoga Class

Because yoga is first approached through a yoga class environment it is necessary to discuss the primary elements involved in an Oriental yoga style class that a student may attend. This chapter can then serve both students to become more aware of what to expect from a class and provide the reasons behind some of the practices. It also aims to serve yoga teachers and instructors in how to conduct an Oriental yoga style class.

Warm up

Warming up the body is a very important part of the practice and cannot be underrated or ignored. Often warming up is overlooked, as modernized man tends to think himself or herself to be time poor. Warming up is essential in calming the energies of the mind, calming the breath and re-establishing a smooth flow of Qi and blood throughout the body. One of the primary aims of warming up is to produce a calming effect, for when the body and nervous system is calmed, the energies of the body flow more easily, which enhances any further practice. 20-30 minutes is the minimal time recommended for gentle warm up practices

Joint release

There are around 300 joints in the human body of which 7 are of primary importance. The 7 primary joints are the:

- Ankles
- Knees
- Hips

- Shoulders
- Elbows
- Wrists and
- Neck

A joint is defined as a place where two bones come to meet. Bones are not designed to have direct contact with each other and are therefore always separated slightly by cartilage, connective tissues, fibrous tissues and fluids that are designed to act like shock absorbers while also supporting the variety of movement of these joints. Keeping this cartilage and fibrous tissue healthy and hydrated is one of the main benefits of a good diet and most yoga practices.

Joints are venerable areas of the body where Qi and blood often become stagnant. A stagnation in Qi and blood in the joints often leads to pain related symptoms and a weakness in the musculature of the area which commonly gives rise to injury. Therefore joint release exercises are of primary importance and at least a few of the primary joints should always be incorporated into any warm up sequence. The following are some instructions for releasing the joints.

Ankles

1. When laying down on your back, gently start to rotate the ankles in circular motions.
2. Avoid going to 100% of you capacity, instead opt for 60-70% only.
3. Focus on smooth movements rather then large movements.
4. After a minute start to move in the other direction.
5. After another minute. Release and shake.

Knees

1. In standing, bring both feet and knees together. Place your hands on your knees and start to do circles with the knees. Again got to only 60-70% of your capacity.
2. After a minute change the direction of the circles.
3. After another minute, stand to release and have a shake.

Hips

1. In standing, bring your hands to your hips. Feet are hip width apart.
2. Start to gently move the hips in a circular motion. Again, sticking to only 60-70% of your capacity. Focus on getting the circles smooth.
3. After a minute, move in the other direction.
4. When completed, stand back into neutral position and release the arms.

Shoulders

1. In standing, gently draw the shoulders forward, then up, then back and then down. Stick to 60-70% of your capacity.
2. Repeat the movement at least 5-10 times, focusing on getting the movement smoother and smoother. If there is any sharp pains then you are going to strong so make the circles much smaller.
3. After 5-10 rounds move in the opposite direction.
4. When done, relax your shoulder and have a shake.

Elbows & Wrists

I have brought these two together because any movement through the wrist naturally affects the elbow joint.

1. In standing, interlace the fingers and gently roll the hands in a circular type motion. Again, keep to only 60-70% of your capacity.
2. After a minute move in the opposite direction.
3. Next, keep the fingers interlaced but this time, bring the elbows out to the side like you're resting your hands and forearms on a desk that is at chest height.
4. Then start to create a wave like motion through the arms and wrists (I call lit the 80's wave dance move). Do this for about a minute.
5. After a minute try and do the wave in the opposite direction.
6. After a minute, release and relax the arms down by your sides.

Neck

With these neck joint releases, do not move to 100% of your capacity! Only go 60-70% of your capacity at all times.

1. In standing, gently start to do circles through the neck with the chin coming forwards slightly and then around to one side, up towards the sky a little bit and then back to the other side. Continue to make gentle circles with the neck in this way. Again, focus on the smoothness of the movement over the size of the movement.
2. After a minute change directions.
3. After a minute in both directions, release and relax.

1. When laying down on your back you can do something very similar to the standing. Gently make circles with your chin. Allow the chin to move towards your chest, over to one side, then up towards the sky and then over to the other side.
2. Continue to make circles in one direction for about a minute and then change directions.
3. When done, release, relax and let your head find its new position.

Pranayama

Pranayama is the movement of Qi throughout the body using the movement of breath. There are potentially hundreds of different pranayama techniques found in yoga, however, in Oriental yoga there is not a great deal of importance placed on practicing any particular pranayama techniques. Rather the importance is placed not on any particular manipulation of breath but rather on developing a natural, efficient and mindful breath that automatically comes about through ongoing practices in asana, relaxation and meditation.

The ideal breathing for a human is to breathe a majority of the time through the nose. Resting the tip of the tongue on the top of the mouth, when at rest and not engaged in any activity using the mouth helps to support the flow of breathe through the nose. Placing the tongue in this position also help to relax the jaw and balances the skull more effectively on the spine. Breathing through the nose has a number of benefits over mouth breathing. They include:

- Warms and filters the air more sufficiently by the time it reaches the lungs
- Supports the slowing of breath and the calming of the nervous system
- Helps to stabilize the Ph levels in the blood
- Reduces the chances of snoring and sleep apnea during sleep
- Increases our sense of smell by keeping the nerves in the nose active and stimulated
- Increases elasticity and strength of the lung tissues due to having a greater resistance of air pressure
- Helps to contain and distribute energy around the body
- Helps to keep the mind sharp and alert

It also helps to balance the skull on the top of the spine and reduces unnecessary strain on the musculature of the face and neck.

In many cases in the modernized human, there is a tendency to over breathe. Meaning that they inhale too much and don't exhale enough. This disturbs the overall body physiology that triggers an inflammatory response and gives rise to respiratory problems such as asthma. Therefore, conditions like asthma are treatable and curable through practices like yoga.

Anxiety related conditions are also mostly triggered by inefficient breathing methods. Through the act of efficient breathing the energies of the mind can easily be tamed and subdued by developing a deeper, slower and more efficient breath.

In meditation and relaxation you will notice the breath will change its rhythm naturally over time and therefore a recommended approach is just to let it re-organize itself without the use of manipulation, but rather, patience.

It is beneficial and advisable to learn efficient and proper breathing at a young age as this will tone up one's overall life force, strengthen the muscles associated with the mechanics of breathing and will also likely give rise to a more vibrant and energized person in adult life. Efficient and proper breathing can be developed at a young age through activates like swimming and learning to play any wind instruments.

Sound

Big sighs, "arrrh," and natural human sounds during the yoga practice are always encouraged and promoted in Oriental yoga due to their powerful affects on deepening the breath, calming the mind and releasing emotional and psychological stressors.

Mantras are useful tools that also help to deepen the breath, release tension and they tend to neutralize the activity of the mind. Essentially, it does not matter which mantra one focuses on and practices because they all produce similar results. However, I have found the following mantras to be simple, effective and of great personal benefit.

On Mani Padme Hum
Nam Myoho Renge Kyo
The Heart Sutra
Hum Saa

Qi Gong

Qi Gong loosely translates as "energy work" and refers to the practice of moving and invigorating Qi energy in and around the body. Qi Gong provides a gentle yet powerful energetic practice that can be incorporated alongside yoga asana practices. Qi Gong could be considered a yin style practice and yoga asana, a yang style practice therefore, both work well to compliment each other.

The main benefits of Qi Gong include:
- Gentle on the joints
- Lubricates and nourishes joints
- Encourages dynamic and proper energy flow
- Supports proper breathing
- Generates sensitivity to the sensation of feeling Qi
- Very calming and relaxing for the nervous system
- Supports the re-training and reorganization of the nervous system and muscle movement behavior for far greater efficiency and effectiveness

Learning the movements of Qi Gong takes some practice and getting used to because it's a completely new way of moving the body. Therefore, for many people it takes a few months of regular class practice to start "getting it" or "feeling it." So, it is fair to say that what we can learn of Qi Gong movements from a book such as this one, is limited. However, I feel it is important to cover some of the basics of Qi Gong because it is an integral part of Oriental Yoga and overall energy training.

A few fundamental principles of Qi Gong are:

- Always keep the joints soft and slightly rounded (do not lock out the joints) as this allows Qi to move easily through these areas.
- Only go 60-90% of one's capacity. Do not over exert as this can drain Qi.
- Synchronize the movement of breath and the movement of the body as one
- Pay attention to the process of movement itself and not to the end position
- It is a continuous movement, never ceasing or stopping unless instructed otherwise
- Move like water, using visualizations of nature and animals are encouraged
- Take your time, for nature does not rush
- Eventually, the movements will happen on their own without any thought required

You can incorporate Qi Gong movements into your practice at any time, e.g. At the beginning of a class, as soon as you wake up, at the end of a class or anytime you feel tired or anxious.

Video media provides a better vehicle for learning the basic movements of Qi Gong than what I can show you through this book. Therefore, I recommend going online and visiting YouTube. Search for "Qi Gong for Beginners" to get access to a number free videos that will show you some basic Qi Gong movements that you can begin to practice. Ideally, enroll into a series of Qi Gong or Tai Chi classes in your area to gain one on one instruction from an experienced practitioner.

Asana

The practice of yoga asanas (postures) serves a variety of purposes. To obtain advanced physical flexibility is not the primary aim in Oriental yoga and does not indicate an advanced yoga practice. More important than physical flexibility is the overall smooth distribution of Qi, blood and the capacity for one to remain mentally equanimous (stable, balanced, unmoving) in the presence of both pleasant and unpleasant sensations that are triggered by yoga asanas.

Asanas serve the following purposes:

1. To support and tone the Qi, blood and overall life force of the practitioner
2. To keep the physical body healthy and posture balanced therefore reducing unnecessary illness and suffering
3. To reduce physical distractions when engaged in meditation
4. To trigger the release of suppressed feelings and emotions that have been stored in the tissues of the body
5. To cultivate inner qualities of focus, attention and determination

Meditation & Contemplation

Traditional meditation in the formal sense refers to sitting quietly and engaging in some kind of mental technique of attention. One of the main benefits of formal meditation practice is the development of concentration. When the mind and attention become concentrated it is much easier for the mind to penetrate any task it is given and therefore provides the foundation for any further mental based training.

Meditation in the informal sense refers to a way of being in the world that is grounded in moment-to-moment awareness. When one is new to meditation, it is recommended to engage firstly in the more formal practices of meditation as these serve to train the nervous system to get more familiar with this state of being. Once this way of being becomes more established in our system, it becomes a more common occurrence to be able to go about our daily activities while in a state of meditation and moment-to-moment awareness.

Contemplation is different to meditation in the sense that one studies or observes certain texts, insight or sayings from verified saints or scripture. The practitioner than simply holds a particular phrase, or a particular line from a sacred text in one's mind for some time. The aim of the practice is for a re-contextualization to occur in the perception of the practitioner so that eventually the truth of that particular phrase or line of sacred text is fully revealed. Contemplation does not mean to intellectualize or think through something, but rather it is more about holding something in mind and allowing it space to "cook." For effective contemplation, one must have some level of concentration and space, so that one is able to continue to cook on one thing at a time, for extended periods if necessary. If the mind is full and mental energies are scattered, contemplation is not very effective and therefore more formal meditational practice may be suitable until one has cultivated a greater capacity for concentration.

Yoga for the Seasons

Part 2

*"Forget the years, forget distinctions.
Leap into the boundless and make it your home!"*

~ *Chuang Tzu*

Earth Element

~ Late Summer ~

Spleen and Stomach

Let's start with the Earth element. The Earth element color is yellow and the season is Late Summer. Lets have a look at an illustration of the 5 elements to see where the Earth element sits within this dynamic play.

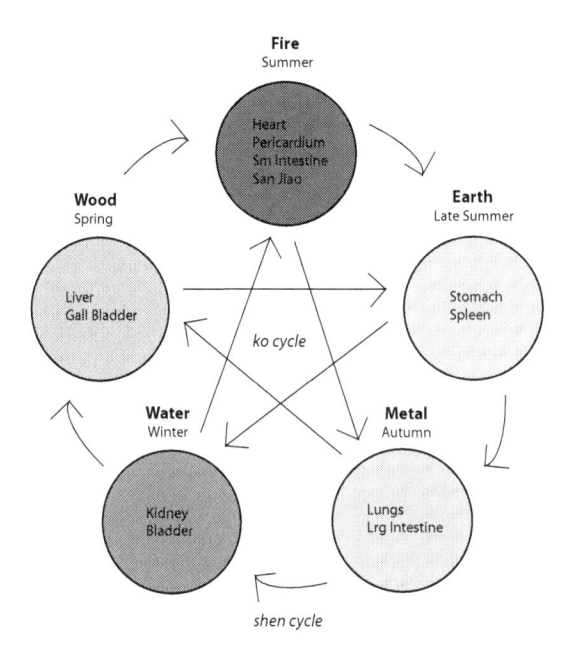

Figure 1.3

When we look at figure 1.3, we can see that the Earth element is supported by the Fire element in the *Shen* (nurturing) cycle and the Wood element supports Earth in the *Ko (controlling)* cycle. I will talk a little more about the Fire element and Wood element later on.

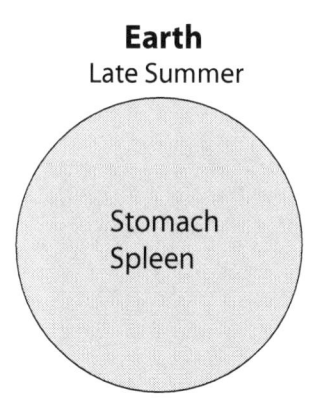

Earth
Late Summer

Stomach
Spleen

Late summer (Earth element) is the most humid time of year. It's that time when the days are still long and hot but the intensity of the summer heat has started to back off a little. In many of the tropical countries it gives rise to the monsoon season. This time of year is closely associated with the digestive organs of the stomach and spleen. Because of the spleen's tendency to enjoy sweet foods there is a natural attraction towards eating sweet, juicy fruit like mangoes and watermelons during this time. The stomach and spleen's internal environment is quite damp, and keeping the internal environment from drying out or from becoming too wet and damp can be a difficult balance to achieve. If the internal environment of the stomach and spleen becomes too dried out the body tends to become excessively skinny and the muscles become thin and weak. On the other hand, if they become too wet and damp, the body becomes excessively overweight, heavy and slow.

The emotions associated with the Earth element are sympathy and empathy as the natural tendency of a mother to a child. Because of the abundance of fruit and vegetables at this time of year, it's time to spend more time in the kitchen cooking, storing and conserving the bountiful harvest for the cooler months ahead.

Late summer is time to get <u>grounded, nourished and feel the support of Mother Earth and the universal life force.</u>

Earth Organ Physiology

Let's have a look at these organs' functions from both a Western medical perspective and an Oriental medical perspective. In most cases, they are both very similar; the main difference being that Oriental medicine adds an energetic and psychological component to the organs.

The spleen in Oriental medicine actually refers to the overall spleen system, which includes the pancreas as well as the spleen.

Stomach function (Western Medicine)

- Receives food from the esophagus
- Stomach secretes acids and enzymes to aid digestion
- Muscles (rugae) line the stomach and contract periodically to churn the food
- A valve called the pyloric sphincter opens to release the churned up food into the small intestine for the next stage of digestion

Spleen Function (Western Medicine)

- Involved in supporting many other organs in the body
- Acts primarily as a filter of blood which supports the immune system
- Replaces blood cells, platelets and stores white blood cells

Pancreas Function (Western Medicine)

- Has two primary functions: a digestive gland and an endocrine gland.
- Produces and secretes important enzymes into the small intestine for digestion
- Produces and secretes hormones insulin and glucagon into the bloodstream to regulate blood glucose levels

Stomach Function (Oriental Medicine)

- Receiving and ripening of food
- Controls digestion of food and water
- Begins the separation of pure from impure—pure goes to storage; impure goes to waste
- Sends the energy downwards
- Keeps digestive system moist, damp and warm for optimal digestive function

Spleen (and Pancreas) Function (Oriental Medicine)

- Governs transportation and transformation of food into blood and Qi and transports it around the body
- Controls the blood and keeps it circulating to the limbs and muscles to keep them healthy and strong
- Stores and excretes urine
- Keeps appetite strong, healthy and regular
- Allows and supports clear thinking and direction
- Keeps you grounded and feeling supported by earth

Physical, Emotional & Spiritual Signs and Symptoms (Oriental medicine)

A Person with Stomach & Spleen In Balance

- Has good healthy digestion
- Good digestive fire (easy to digest foods)

- Feels energized after eating
- Eats without distractions (no phones, computers, TV or newspapers). Chews slowly and with awareness. Often offering a prayer of gratitude before and after meals
- Eats at the same time every day (great way to restore balance)
- Has good muscle tone and strong limbs
- Can think clearly, has the ability to stay focused for long periods
- Ability to feel sympathy and empathy towards others without giving out and losing energy
- Feels centered, grounded, confident, strong and able
- Has trust in the universe (does not worry about future)
- Feels supported and nourished by Mother Earth (bountiful)
- Enjoys community, connections and is generous
- Has a strong sense of identity yet understands that one is included in a greater picture therefore doesn't exhibit self-centeredness, selfishness or self-absorption
- Enjoys moving and exercising the body because it increases their capacity to feel stable, strong, focused and centered
- Wakes up early, takes time to ground and integrate, getting ready for the day
- Peaks workflow at 9-11am
- Able to relax and sleep well at night

Stomach and Spleen Out Of Balance

With an imbalance in these organs you can either experience the extreme of having too much fire energy and not enough fluids (drying up) or on the other extreme, and more commonly, not enough fire energy and too many fluids, which allows the digestion to become too damp and heavy.

- Always worrying, especially about an uncertain future
- Over thinks, talks more than does
- Over plans things, needs to plan well in advance

- Ungrounded, unclear, very "flighty", unstable, inability to focus for extended periods (commonly shows ADD and ADHD symptoms)
- Doesn't eat enough protein and replaces the lack of proper nutrition with processed sugars to get energy bursts
- Poor appetite; often doesn't eat breakfast and eats at irregular times
- Thin, colorless lips
- Eats while at working desk, watching TV or reading something
- Heartburn, nausea, vomiting and burps often after meals (energy flowing upward instead of downward)
- Lacks muscle tone, weak limbs
- Overweight (too much damp) or underweight (too hot and dry)
- Poor sluggish digestion (too much damp) or overactive digestion (too hot and dry) with an inability to put on weight
- Feelings of a heavy body
- Ongoing constipation or diarrhea
- Gets colds and flu easily
- Unable to sympathize or empathize with others
- Often self-absorbed and self-centered
- Unable to trust others or the universe; always worried!
- Often manifests as type 2 diabetes
- Lacks sense of community and dislikes sharing with others (self focused)
- Feels tired after meals

The main causes of imbalance are due to an over abundance of sweetened foods (processed sugars), a tendency towards excessive worry and not enough physical movement or training. This is very common in the Western world and is now becoming more common in the East as people are taking to sweetened foods and spending extended times on computers and sitting in chairs. Later, we will discuss how to bring this common imbalance back into balance. It's not difficult to address this imbalance but it does take time and a change in priorities, but it can add years to your life and installs a strong sense of self responsibility, groundedness and stability in one's life.

The Earth Element Meridians

Earth is directly associated with the stomach and spleen organs and meridians, so let's have a look at these meridians and where they travel.

Stomach Meridian

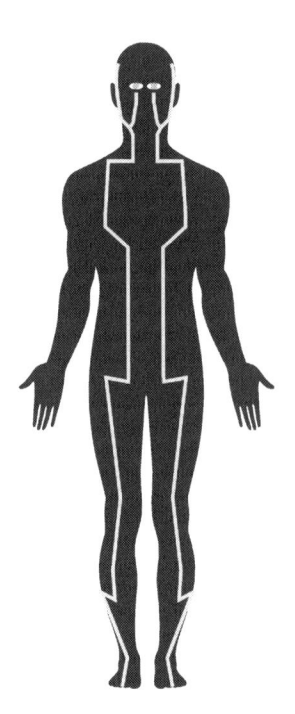

The stomach channel begins just below the centre of both eyes. It then moves down through the gums and heads out to the jaw. One branch heads up to the side of the forehead passing the front of the ear; the other branch heads down the front of the throat to the collarbone region. A branch then travels internally to meet the organs of the stomach and spleen while another superficial branch travels down the front of the body, over the abdomen and down the to pubic area. The internal branch and the superficial branch re-join at the public area and the channel continues down the front of the thigh and down the outside of the kneecap. The channel continues to descend down the top of the foot and finishes at the middle toe.

Spleen Meridian

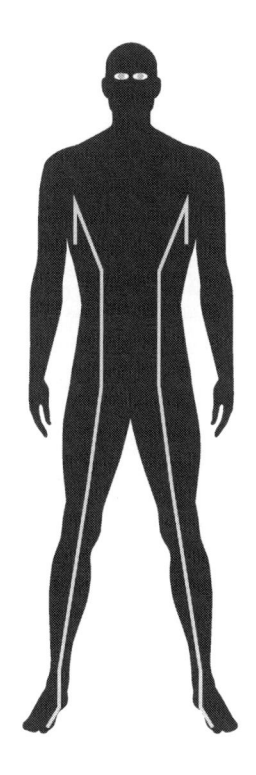

The Spleen channel begins on the inside tip of the big toe. It travels up the inside of the foot and continues up the inside of the ankle and inner leg. It continues up the inside of the leg to the groin where it briefly travels internally. It resurfaces for a short time on the lower abdomen where it then returns inside to meet up with the spleen, stomach, diaphragm and heart. A branch continues up the inside of the body to the tongue. The superficial branch travels up the side of the chest and then descends to a place in the rib cage under the armpit.

Muscles Associated with the Stomach

The recommended asanas are explored in the next chapter, but first let's get a little more familiar with the muscles directly associated with the stomach.

Anterior Neck Flexors and Extensors

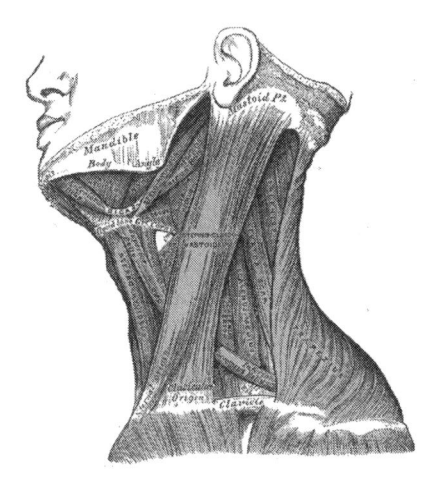

There are many muscles in the neck area that control neck flexion or extension. Generally, all the muscles in the front of the neck are called anterior neck flexors and assist in the movement of drawing the head forward. All the muscles at the back of the neck are considered neck extensors and work to draw the head back. Ideally, both neck flexors and extensors work as a synchronized team to balance the head and keep the spine aligned. In many cases, one set of muscles is overworked and in a state of tension whereas the other set of muscles are weak and not very active or strong. An indicator of an imbalance in these groups of muscles in the neck is ongoing sinus problems.

Brachioradialis

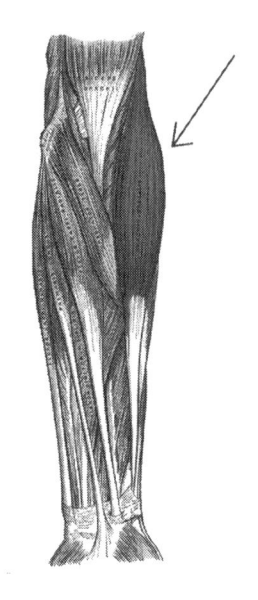

The picture above is of a left arm in anterior view, meaning it's showing the inside of the arm with the left thumb on the side of the brachioradialis muscle that has the arrow directed at it. The muscle originates on the lateral supercondylar ridge of the humerus and attaches to the styloid process of the radius. Its main action is to flex the arm at the elbow (drawing the hand up). Therefore it could be said that people with strong forearm muscles would likely have good digestion.

Lavater Scapulae

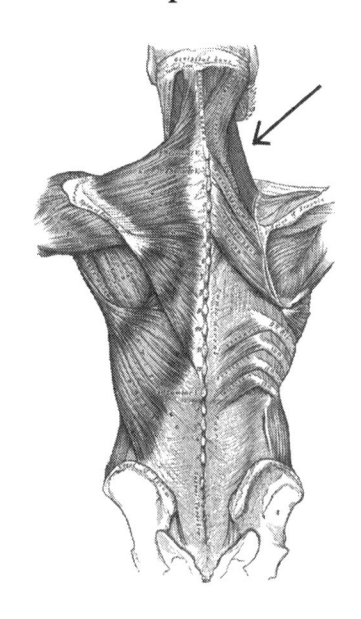

This muscle originates deep in the neck and is attached to the transverse processes of cervical vertebrae one to four. The muscle then travels down to the shoulder area and attaches to the medial border of the scapula.

Muscles Associated with the Spleen

Most of the muscles associated with the spleen are in the back of the body and indicate that healthy back muscles also support a healthy digestive system as well as a healthy spine.

Latissimus Dorsi

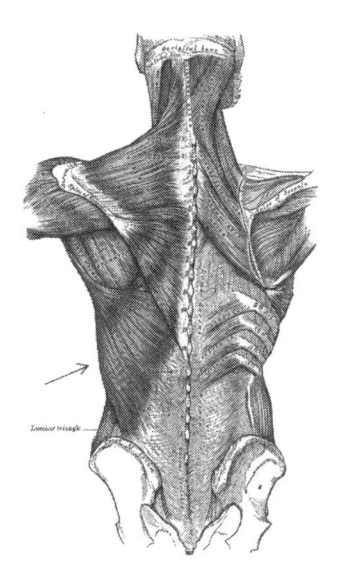

The Latissimus Dorsi is a powerful muscle in the lower and middle back. It originates at a number of different locations—the lumber vertebrae, the lower six thoracic vertebrae, the iliac crest, the sacrum, the lower 3 or 4 ribs and the inferior angle of the scapula. It wraps around the lower and middle back to attach itself to the inertubercular groove of the humerus.

Middle & Lower Trapezius

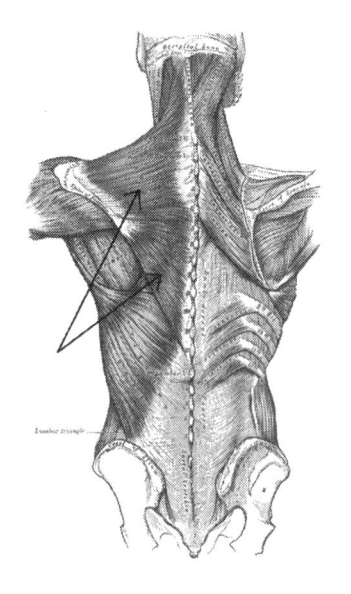

This picture shows the whole trapezius muscle. It can be broken down into the upper, middle and lower trapezius. The middle trapezius originates at the spinous process of C7, T1, T2 & T3 and attaches to the medial and upper border of the scapula. The lower trapezius originates from the spinous process of T4-T12 and attaches to the inferior medial border of the scapula.

Triceps Brachii

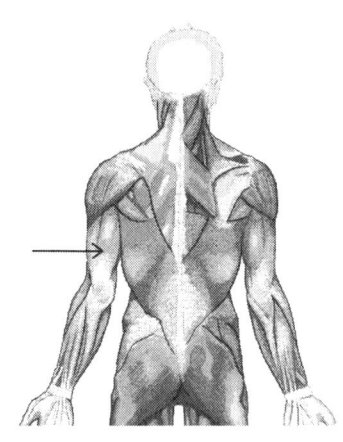

The triceps are known as the "3 headed arm muscle" due to the muscle having 3 different origin points. The longest head of muscle originates from the infraglenoid tubercle of the scapula. The middle head originates from the dorsal surface of the humerus and the third head originates in close proximity to the middle head as it also originates on the back of the humerus bone from the greater tubercle down to the region of the lateral intermuscular septum.

Opponens Pollicis Longus

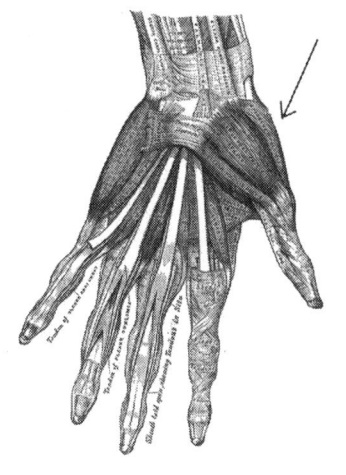

This muscle is found on in the inside of the palm and acts to flex the thumb towards the little finger. It originates on the tubercle of the trapezium bone and the flexor retinaculum and inserts onto the anterior and lateral surfaces of the shaft of the first metacarpal bone.

Asanas (Postures) for Late Summer

The main aim with the late summer asana practices is to open the stomach and spleen channels on the front of the body, while strengthening and toning the muscles around the spine on the back of the body. Cultivating power and strength in the legs also helps to ground the system's energy into the earth. The following pages explore some asanas that achieve this aim.

Incorporate these postures into your asana practice during late summer to stimulate the stomach and spleen.

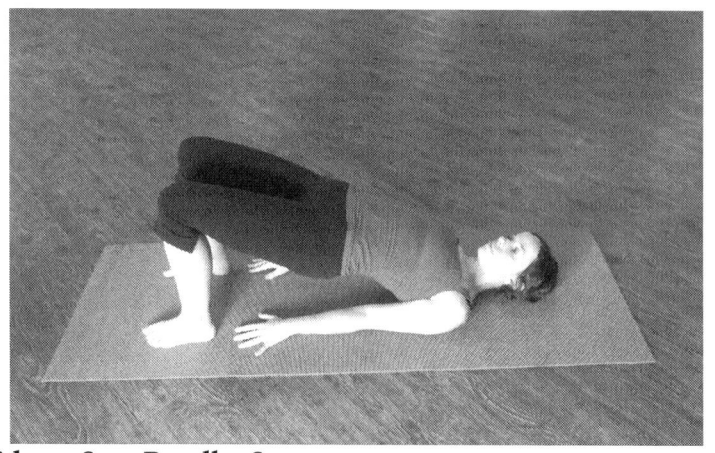

Bridge – Setu Bandha Sarvangasana
Main benefit – Strengthens the back muscles and opens the front of the body.

1. Lie on your back on the mat, arms along the side of the body, palms down.

Oriental Yoga

2. Bend your knees, place your feet on the mat close to your buttocks, feet hip width apart.
3. As you inhale, flatten your back into the mat and as you exhale, slowly peel your hips from the floor and push them towards the sky.
4. When you reach the top, suck your belly in, look down the midline of your body with your head still on the floor. Work the arms and hands gently into the floor and gently squeeze the knees towards each other. The knees do not need to touch; the inner thighs just need to be activated.
5. Find your breath and hold for at least three long breaths.
6. When you are ready, inhale to rise a little higher, then, as you exhale, start to slowly peel your spine back onto the mat. Rest.
7. Repeat this action 2-3 times.

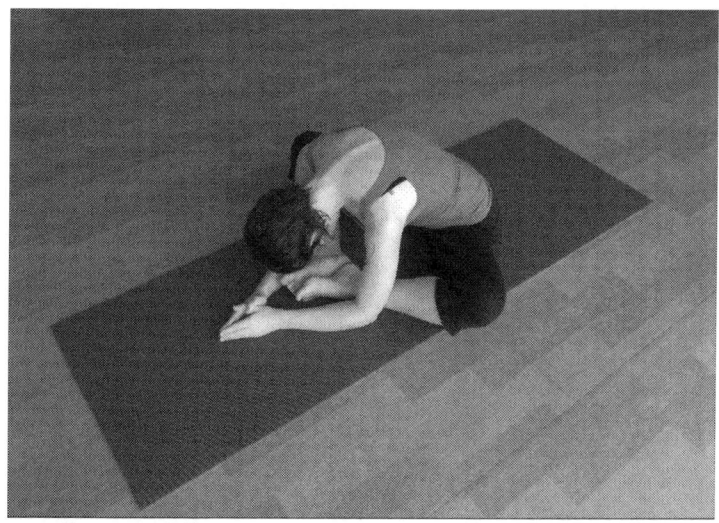

Butterfly – Buddha Konasana
Main benefit – Opens the inner legs and opens the back of the body.

1. Sitting on the floor or on some folded blankets, bring the soles of your feet together. Give yourself some space between your groin and your feet.

2. Grabbing hold of your feet, inhale to lengthen the spine; exhale to draw your heart space down toward your feet and the floor.
3. Allow yourself to move into this pose slowly. While deep in the pose, really focus on relaxing your legs and knees toward the floor. Relax your back and draw your head toward the floor, relaxing the back of your neck and shoulder. Close your eyes and breathe here for a few minutes.
4. When you're ready to come up, simply roll up slowly back into a sitting position with your back straight.

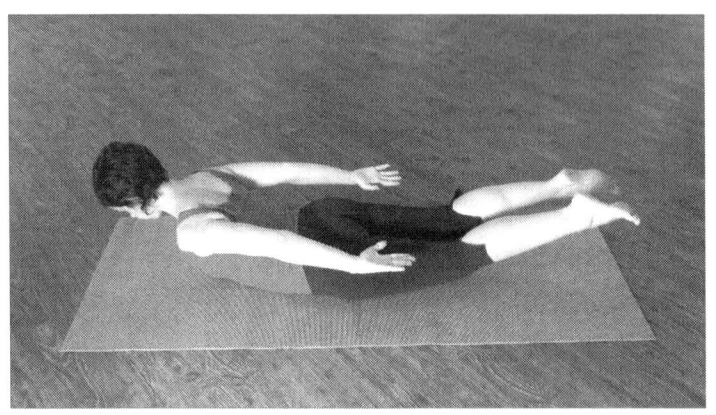

Locust - Salabhasana
Main benefit – Strengthens the back of the body which includes the neck extensors.

1. Lie on your belly in the middle of your mat.
2. Bring the arms down the side of the body, palms facing up. Feet hip width apart. Looking forward, resting the head on the chin.
3. On an inhale, start to raise the upper body, the arms and hands off the floor. Try to get the arms parallel with the floor.
4. Then start to raise the legs off the floor. Try to keep your legs straight.
5. Look diagonally down towards the floor to keep the neck in line with the spine.

6. Now gently squeeze the hands towards each other so you activate the muscles around the shoulder blades.
8. Keep the breath moving. Hold for 3-4 breaths and then slowly release and relax back onto your mat.
9. Have a little rest for a few moments and do it at least one more time.

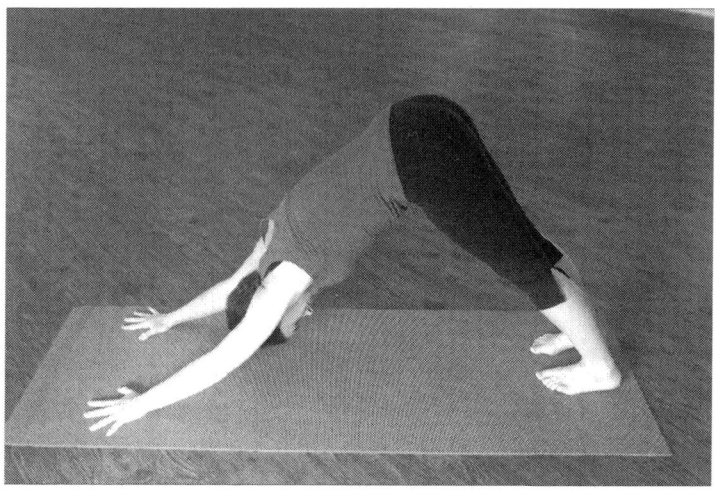

Down Facing Dog – Adho Mukha Svanasana
Main benefit – Strengthens arms, shoulders and opens the back of the legs.

1. Come onto all fours with hands underneath the shoulders and knees under the hips. Spread your fingers wide.
2. Tuck the toes under, start to extend the arms and start bringing the knees off the floor
3. Come to extend the arms and start to work the legs straight. Try to bring the weight back into your legs and not so much into your arms.
4. Look to the floor just under your belly button.

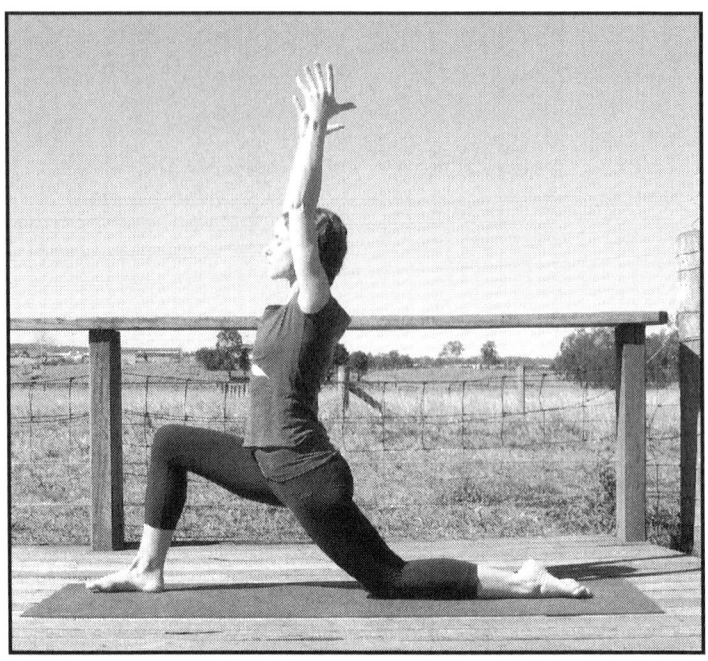

Low Lunge – Anjaneyasana

Main benefit – Opens the psoas muscle, the front of the body, and strengthens the back.

1. Ideally, you will start in a standing-forward, bent position (Uttanasana) at the front of the mat. Then simply step your left leg to the back of the mat and bring your back knee to the floor; the top of your back foot should be flat on the floor.
2. Make sure your front ankle is either just in front of or directly underneath your front knee.
3. Open your heart up and bring your arms out to the side, and then bring them up above your head. In this picture, the hands are shoulder width apart—this makes it easier to relax the shoulders down away from the ears. You can bring your hands together too, if that feels more natural.
4. Allow your lower back to lengthen and gently work your hips forward and down toward the floor, opening the front of your left hip.

5. After a few breaths, bring your torso and your arms down toward the floor, tuck your back toe under and step to the front of the mat, returning to your forward bend at the front of the mat.
6. Repeat on the other side.

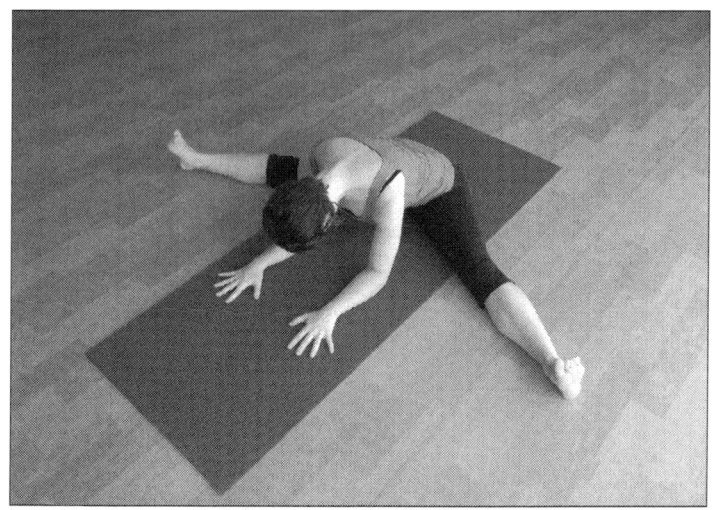

Wide Legged Seated Forward Bend – Upavistha Konasana
Main benefit – Opens the inside of the legs

1. Start by sitting on the floor or upon some folded blankets (recommend the folded blankets for this one).
2. Bring your legs out wide—to about 90% of your capacity.
3. Start by bringing your hands onto the floor behind your back. Inhale to lengthen your spine and draw your toes back; exhale to use your arms to draw your torso forward and down.
4. If you are new to this stretch then it is probably best to keep your hands behind your back to help you out. If you are more flexible, then bring your hands out in front of your body and use them to help you forward and down.
5. Take your time with this one. Use your breath to support you. You can experiment a little with this one by moving your torso

slightly to the left or right to get a different kind of stretch in your inner legs. Stay as long as you like.
6. When ready to come out, simply draw yourself up back into a seated position and slowly draw your legs together.

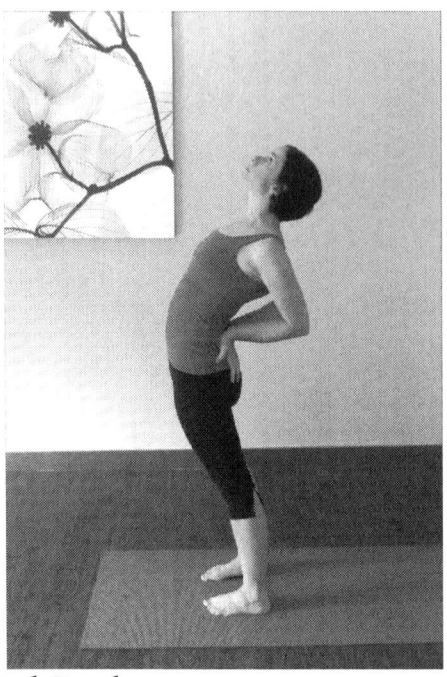

Standing Back Bend
Main Benefit –Strengthens the back of body and opens the front.

1. Place your hands, onto the lower back with finger pointing downwards.
2. Draw the elbows towards each other; suck the belly in before gently drifting the hips forward and leaning back.
3. Feel the heart and throat open. Only hold for a breath and then come out.
4. Come out by drawing your torso forward and releasing the arms. Feel free to move the hips around in circles to release and then try again.

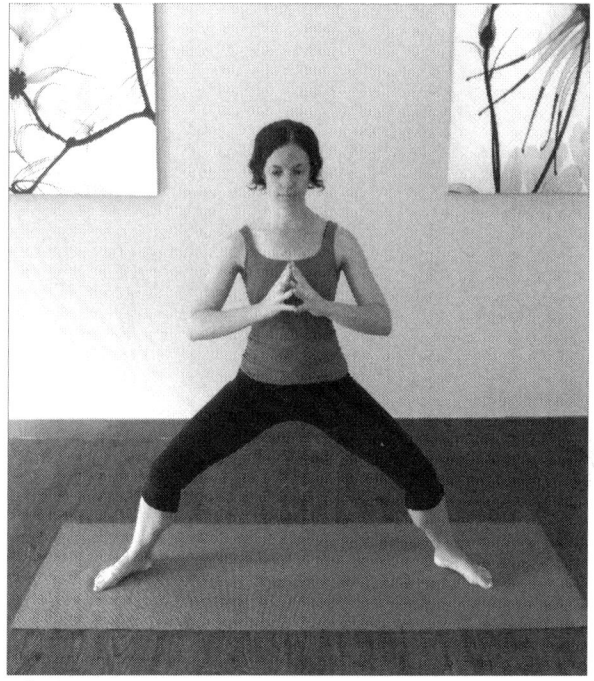

Horse Stance
Main benefit – Strengthens and grounds the legs into the earth.

1. Stand in the centre of your mat
2. Bring your legs wide apart (about 1 leg's length apart)
3. Bring your hands into prayer position; relax the shoulders, arms are light.
4. Start to gently squat into your legs, keep the knees working back so you're working the hips open.
5. Once you find a spot where you feel "switched on" and activated through the legs, hold it for some time.
6. Connect with your breath. Gently squeeze Mula Bundha (gentle squeeze of the anus muscle) and hold the posture.
7. Hold for at least 10 long steady breaths before slowly easing up and coming out of it.
8. Be sure to practice this a few times in each session. It's a great practice to do if you feel too "heady".

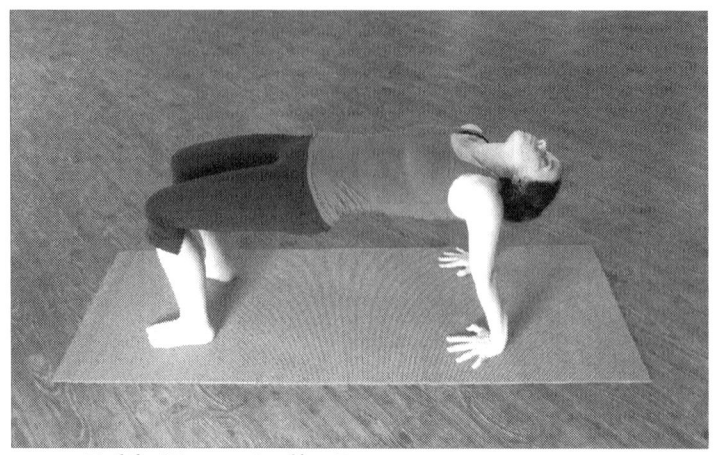

Reverse Table Top – Ardha Purvottanasana
Main Benefit – Strengthens the back of the body and opens the front.

1. Come to sit on your mat, with your knees bent and feet flat on the mat.
2. Bring your hands just behind you, fingers pointing forwards.
3. Start by raising the buttocks just off the floor.
4. If ok, raise the hips all the way so they are in line with your knees and shoulders.
5. Let your head rest back into the fold of the neck.
6. Get a sense of the shoulder working down away from the head. Allow the elbows to have a tiny bend in them, avoid hyperextending the elbow joint.
7. Plant your fingers and toes into the floor.
8. Connect with your breath and hold for around 5 long steady breaths.
9. To come out slowly, lower your buttocks first; the head will naturally roll up without any effort.
10. Come to sit back on the mat.

Other techniques that stimulate the Stomach and Spleen:

Singing

Have you heard that singing is good for digestion? According to Oriental medicine, singing stimulates Qi and blood while also calming the mind. Therefore, activities like going out to karaoke after dinner or even singing in the shower are a recommended practice, especially in late summer.

Massage the Legs

1. Sit either on the floor or on a comfortable chair and start to gently squeeze the *inside* of one of your lower legs. Work up from the ankle to the knee. The inside of the leg contains the spleen, kidney and liver channels. The inside of the leg is considered to be yin and triggers a relaxed and sometimes sleepy state.

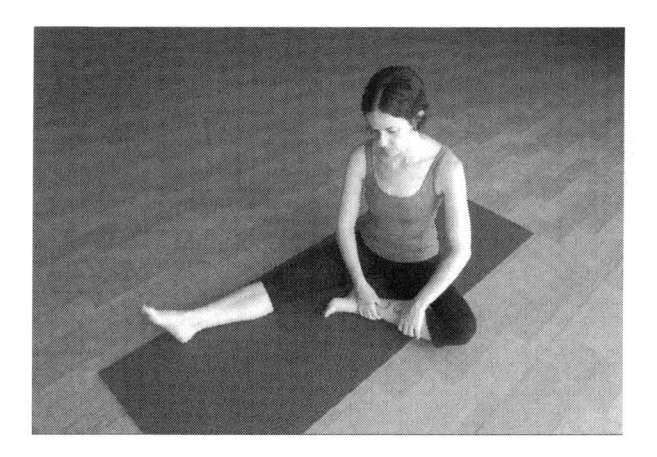

2. After you have worked on the inside of the legs, move your attention to the outside of the legs. Bend one knee up and start to pummel (loose fist thumping) the outside of the lower leg. Work up from above the ankle to around the knee. After a good pummeling, use your palm and thumb to squeeze the muscles on

the outside of the leg. The outside of the leg contains the stomach and gallbladder channels and is considered to be more stimulating and energizing due to it being a yang part of the body.

Mindful Eating and Prayers for Eating

Practicing mindful eating can be one of the most powerful practices to nourish and support the stomach and spleen while also training the mind. Mindful eating involves eating slowly, with full awareness and without distraction. Also, including a little prayer, as a way to give thanks to Mother Earth and as a way to purify the food, is an age-old practice that many spiritual and religious traditions still practice. The following example of a mindfulness food prayer comes from Buddhist monk Thich Nhat Hanh, from his book *Savor: Mindful Eating, Mindful Life*.

The Five Contemplations
1. This food is the gift of the whole universe: The earth, the sky, numerous living beings and much hard, loving work.

2. May we eat with mindfulness and gratitude so as to be worthy to receive it.

3. May we recognize and transform our unwholesome mental formations, especially our greed, and learn to eat with moderation.

4. May we keep our compassion alive by eating in such a way that we reduce the suffering of living beings, preserve our planet and reverse the process of global warming.

5. We accept this food so that we may nurture our sisterhood and brotherhood, strengthen our community, and nourish our ideal of serving all living beings.

Earth Element Daily Lifestyle Practices

- Eat a nourishing, grounding, and protein-fuelled breakfast between 7-9am. Take your time.

- Avoid watching TV, reading newspapers or magazines, looking at your phone or listening to commercial radio when eating food.

- Eat at similar times each day.

- Avoid ice cold drinks.

- Spend more time in the kitchen, cooking, preparing and preserving foods.

- Add ginger to your cooking to stimulate digestion.

- Avoid over thinking or over worrying. If you find yourself falling into that trap, do more physical activity—go for a walk, go to a yoga class, etc. Don't pay so much attention to your thinking mind. Trust the universe that it will all work out okay and go with it.

- Engage in activities that help to build a sense of community. Be generous. Share food.

- Do your biggest thinking tasks, finalizing big decisions and facing difficult clients between 9-11am. Avoid making big decisions in the afternoon or nighttime.

- Do weights and resistance training (morning is best). Resistance/strength training will strengthen your muscles, improve digestion and help you think more clearly.

- Cultivate trust and faith in the natural flow of life. Avoid doubt or over thinking everything—let it unfold naturally, the universe is infinitely organized! Let it do its thing; no need to try and 'work it out' or force it to change.

Supporting the Other Elements to Assist the Earth Element

As outlined in the 5 elements chapter, if we want to balance out the Earth element, we also need to take into consideration the elements that feed the Earth element. This is especially the case if any illness or disease becomes present around the stomach or spleen. The elements that nourish and support the Earth element are the Fire element (*Shen* cycle) and the Wood element (*Ko* cycle).

Fire Element Nourishment

- Add a little chili and spice in your foods to generate more heat in your belly.
- Dream big. Find inspiration. Have fun.
- Arrange inspirational meetings around midday.
- Connect with others who inspire and motivate you.
- Practice meditation to calm the mind and nurture the heart.

Wood Element Stimulation and Harmonization

- Wood element likes to move so keep the body moving to avoid stagnation. Going for a walk can often be enough.
- Reduce or avoid alcohol, coffee, BBQ'd foods and smoking.
- De-clutter your environment and remove the non-essentials.
- Launch into new projects.
- Get to bed before 11pm and wake early.
- Drink lemon water on rising.

Food / Oriental Diet Therapy ~ Late Summer

During *late summer*, the following foods and methods are recommended for nourishing and supporting the organs:

Method of Cooking: Soups, stews, baking and slow cooking

Grains: Whole grains, rice, oats, roasted barley, sweet rice, spelt, miller

Vegetables: Pumpkin, sweet potatoes, squash, carrots, corn, parsnips, yams, peas, onions, leeks, garlic, mushrooms

Beans and Nuts: Chick peas, black beans, kidney beans, fava beans, walnuts

Meat: Small amounts of chicken, beef, lamb, goose, mackerel, tuna, eel, catfish

Herbs and Seasonings: Black pepper, ginger, cinnamon, nutmeg, fennel

Fruit Sugars: Barley malt, dates, figs, cherries, sugar cane

Avoid / Reduce
- Salads
- Raw fruits and raw vegetables
- Citrus

- Wheat
- Refined sugars, chocolate
- Ice-cream, smoothies & ice water
- Alcohol (a little warm wine is ok)

Herbs to Support the Stomach and Spleen

Here is a list of herbs that support the main organs involved in keeping the stomach and spleen healthy. Taking herbs alongside a healthy lifestyle that incorporates yoga will provide more effective results. Just taking herbs without engaging in other supportive methods often brings little results.

Please seek guidance from a health professional (naturopath, herbalist, Chinese herbalist, Chinese medicine practitioner) for more information about correct dosages or for treating specific conditions.

Astragalus - Supports Qi and supports the immune system

Citrus Peel – Supports digestion

Ginger – Warms the digestive system

Wild Cardamom – Warms the digestive system

Dioscorea Oppositifolia (Mountain Yam) – Tones spleen and dries up damp

Chamomile Tea – Dries damp and calms nervous system

Late Summer Meditations

<u>Grounding Meditation</u>

Preparation: Sit in a comfortable position. If you are sitting on the floor, I always recommend sitting up on a folded blanket—ideally, you want your knees to be just below your hips. This will help you sit for longer periods without extra stress in your back. Ok, when you're in a comfortable seated position, place your hands in any comfortable position.

Ok, when you feel steady, close your eyes and settle into a relaxed posture. Find your breath moving through your nostrils and keep watching it. Just keep your attention on your breath, let your mind's content just move through without giving it much attention. Relinquish your mind's thoughts and images as they arise. Come back to your breath with an alert, yet relaxed, awareness. Just watch your breath for at least five minutes until your mind starts to settle.

When your mind has settled a little, move your awareness down to where your buttocks and back of the legs touch the floor. Notice your connection to the floor. Feel the support from the floor. Now, imagine dropping a line, like a sink line used in fishing, from the base of your spine down into the earth, deep into the earth. Hold that image for a number of breaths.

After a number of breaths and the sense of feeling rooted to the earth via the sink line from the base of the spine, draw your attention to your lower belly. Now, as you breathe in, focus your attention on this point and say to yourself, "*Hummmmm*", and as you breathe out, say to yourself, "*Saaaaaaaa*".

Do this for a few minutes.

Next, move your attention to your upper belly area. As you breathe in, focus your attention on this point and say to yourself, "*Hummmmm*", and as you breathe out, say to yourself, "*Saaaaaaaa*".

Do this for a few minutes.

After some time, when you feel ready to move on, begin to visualize a gentle smiling face in your minds eye. Once you have the image, send the smiling face down to the area of your belly. Give thanks to the belly by allowing in the smiling face to spread out and permeate the entire belly area.

To complete this mediation, bring your attention back to your breath at your nostrils. Let go of all other practices. Watch your breath until you feel calm and relaxed. Then, when ready, open your eyes gently and release your posture.

Metal Element

~ Autumn ~

Lung and Large Intestine

Next up is Metal element. Let's have a look at the 5 elements to see where the Metal Element sits within this dynamic play.

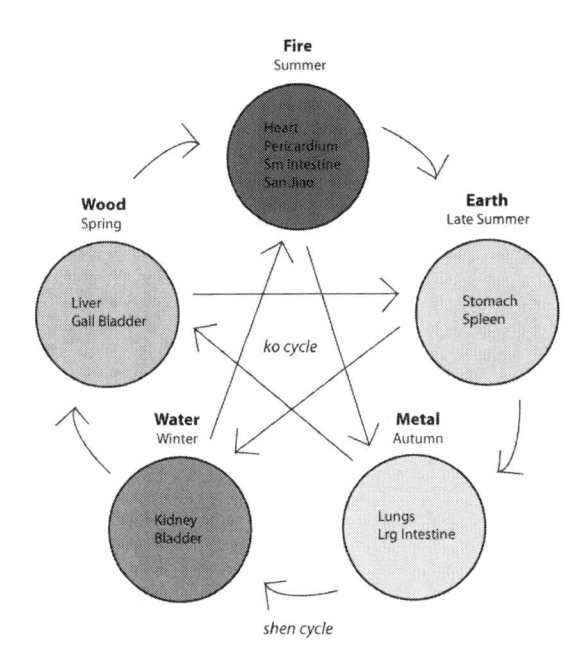

figure 1.3

When we look at figure 1.3 we can see that the Metal Element is supported by the Earth element in the *Shen* (nurturing) cycle and the Fire element supports Metal in the *Ko (controlling)* cycle. I will talk a little more about the Earth element and Fire element later on.

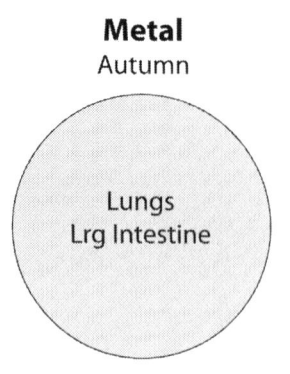

Metal
Autumn

Lungs
Lrg Intestine

Autumn (Metal Element) is the transformational period from the expansive energy of summer to the more introverted energy of winter. Because we are moving away from the energy of summer, it's a time to start slowing things down, time to tie up loose ends, refine ones character and let go of the things, ideas and goals that don't serve us any longer. The organs associated with autumn are the lungs and large intestine. Both these organs play a large part in the detoxification of the body and this is also relevant to the detoxification of the mind - meaning it's a time to let go of any grudges or things that tie us too our past and clear some space for being in the now.

Metal Organ Physiology

Let's have a look at the Lung and Large Intestine functions from both a Western medical perspective and an Oriental medical perspective. Again, in most cases, they are both very similar; the main difference being that Oriental medicine adds an energetic and psychological component to the organs.

Lung function (Western Medicine)

- Detoxification
- Brings O2 into the body and removes Carbon Dioxide
- Gas transportation

Large Intestine Function (Western Medicine)

- Peristalsis (rhythmic muscle contractions)
- Bacterial digestion
- Absorption
- Defecation

Lung Function (Oriental Medicine)

- Controls respiration
- Contributes greatly to the Immune System by spreading out the Qi (defence Qi, immune system) around your body. (The neck area is weak point)
- Controls dispersing and descending of Qi
- Control the skin and hair
- Detoxification
- Opens into the nose

Large Intestine Function (Oriental Medicine)

- Receive waste from small intestine
- Communicates with the Lungs
- Absorbs fluids
- Defecation

Physical, Emotional & Spiritual Signs and Symptoms (Oriental medicine)

Lung & Large Intestine <u>In Balance</u>

- Rarely affected by colds and flues
- Wakes early
- Have regular and healthy bowel movements (not too loose or dry)
- Able to let go of the past and grudges
- Prefers structure and organization
- Quality in work, refinement
- Integrity is very important
- Can access and enjoys the 'present moment'
- Breathes efficiently, deeply and smoothly
- Is affected by grief and sadness but is able to be with it and accept its presence.
- Powerful and pleasant voice
- Healthy skin

Lung & Large Intestine <u>Out Of balance</u>

- Anxiety, shallow breathing, panic attacks
- Self doubt, loss of spiritual connection
- Difficult to relax into the present moment
- Gets cold and flu's easily
- Very dry or loose, wet stools

- Ongoing constipation
- Structure turns into rigidity and stiffness
- Repressed emotions - especially grief, sadness, bitterness, regret
- Unable to let go
- Hoards too much stuff, doesn't throw anything out– attachment to material stuff
- A tendency to be addicted to smoking
- Skin rashes, skin problems, boils, dry skin etc.
- Sinus problems
- Difficult to breath through nose
- Repertory conditions like asthma
- Easy to fatigue
- Sweating (other organs can also involved)

The Metal Element Meridians

Autumn is directly associated with the Lung and Large Intestine organs and meridians, so let's have a look at these meridians and where they travel around the body.

Lung Meridian

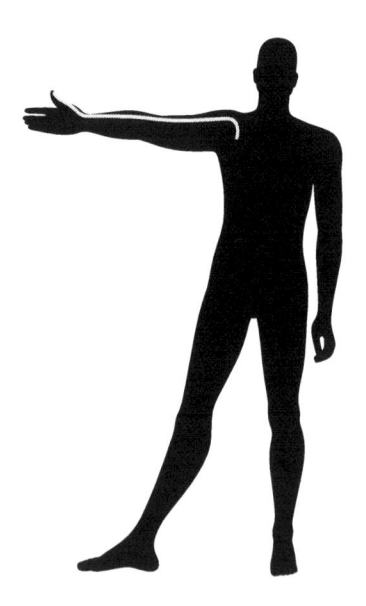

The lung channel begins deep inside the body around the solar plexus area and then moves downwards to meet the large intestine. It then moves upwards through the lungs and into the windpipe. It then divides and moves out towards the arm where it surfaces just under the collarbone. From here it passes over the shoulder and down the front aspect of the arm. It passes just on the outside of the biceps tendon at the elbow crease and continues down the forearm to the wrist. At the base of the thumb it then travels over the thumb muscle to finish at the corner of the thumbnail.

Large Intestine

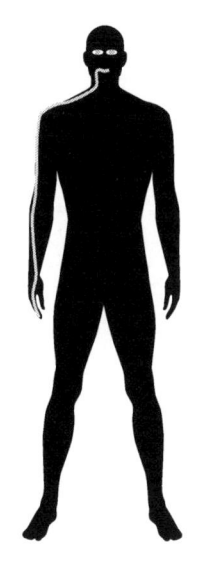

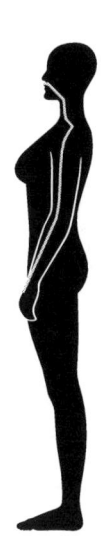

The large intestine meridian begins on the outer edge of the index finger. It then travels along the finger, running up towards the wrist and then up the outside edge of the forearm. It then continues to the outside edge of the elbow crease, which is visible when the arm is bent. Then it travels up the outside edge of the upper arm and across the top of the shoulder and across the top of the shoulder blade. It then descends internally to connect with the lungs and large intestine. A branch continues to travel upwards over the shoulder muscles to the front area of the neck to the cheek and then over the top of the lip. It finishes beside the opposite nostril where it links with the stomach channel.

Muscles Associated with the Lungs

The following are the muscles that are associated with the lung organ and meridian.

Anterior Serratus

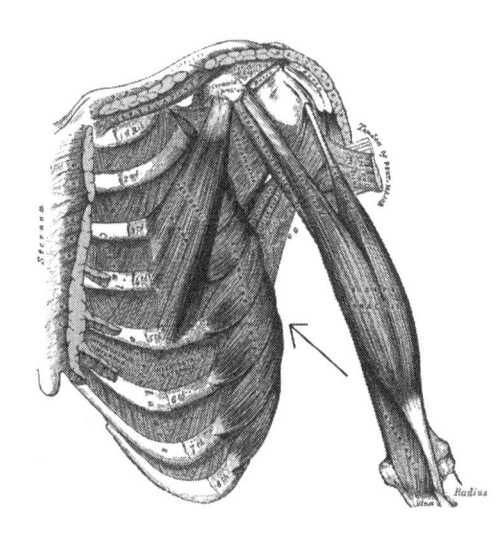

Anterior Serratus are the muscles that originate on the surface of the ribs on the side of the chest and rap around the rib cage and insert onto the medial border of the scapula on the back of the body. You may consider them to be the attachment point of your wings.

They are involved in the raising of the arms above shoulder height. They also help the rib cage to expand and contract when breathing.

Anterior Deltoids

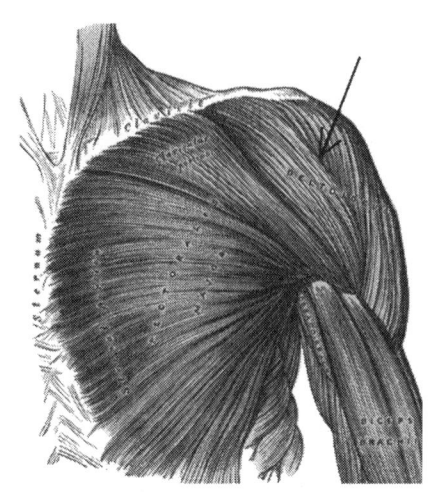

The deltoids are known as the "common shoulder muscle" and form the rounded contour of the shoulder. It is made up of three district set of fibers, one being the on the front of the shoulder (anterior deltoid), one on the outside of the shoulder (lateral deltoid) and the set of fibers at the back of the shoulder (posterior deltoid).

The deltoids are involved whenever we move the arms about. Push up like training will activate the front of the deltoids, while side arm raises will get the outside of the deltoids and any movement with the arms behind the torso will activate the deltoids at the back of the shoulder.

The Diaphragm

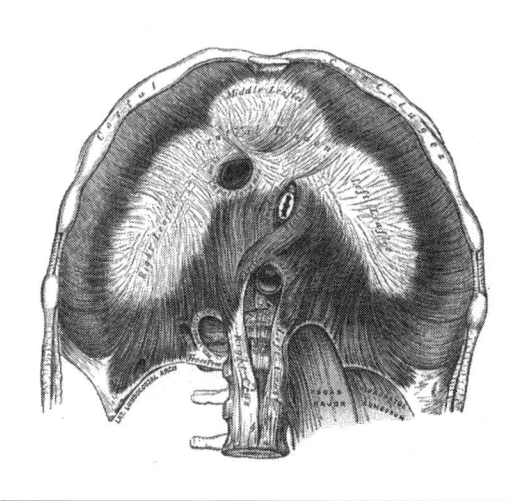

The diaphragm is like a sheet of muscle that separates the thoracic cavity (heart and lungs) from the abdominal cavity. It helps perform the important function of respiration by contracting and increasing the volume of the thoracic cavity so that air is drawn down into the lungs.

It is activated whenever we breathe. We can tone the diaphragm by performing efficient breathing and drawing in the belly slightly when doing yoga asanas.

The picture on the previous page illustrates what it looks like from just below the diaphragm, in the abdominal cavity looking upwards.

Caracobrachialis

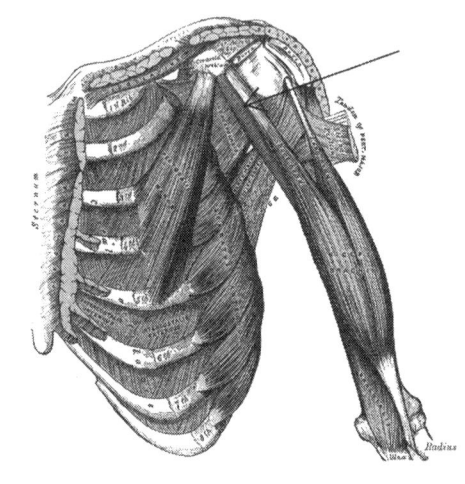

The coracobrachialis is one of the smallest muscles on the front of the shoulder. Its origin is from the apex of the coracoid process and attaches on the medial surface of the humerus.

Situated at the front of the shoulder it is activated any time we have arms out in front of the body, like in the push up position.

Muscles Associated with the Large Intestine

Hamstrings

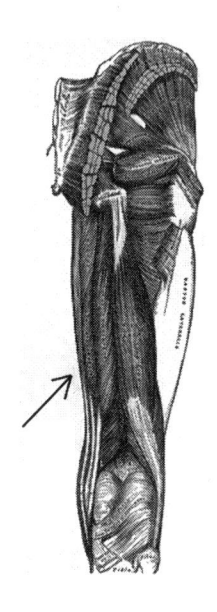

Situated at the back of the upper leg are 3 main muscles that make up the hamstrings. Many people have tight hamstrings, mainly due to sitting in chairs where the hamstrings are always contracted. A lot of anger and similar emotions get stored in the legs and hamstrings.

The hamstrings are activated anytime we bend our knees. They are lengthened when we straighten the legs.

Tensor Fasciae Latae

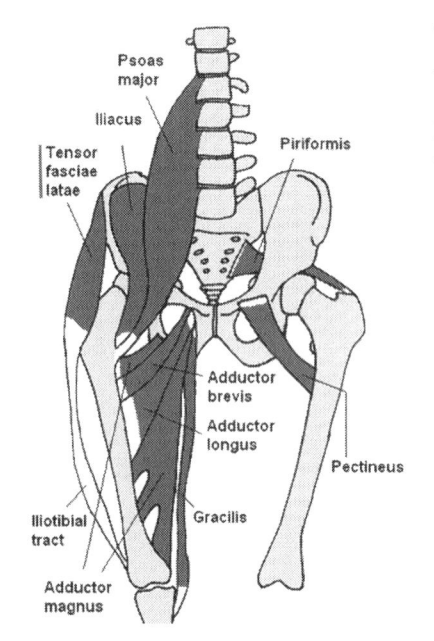

The tensor fasciae latae attaches to the iliac crest and extends itself down the outside of the hip where it attaches to the illiotibial band. It is often very tender and super tight especially in runners or those with tight hips in general.

This little muscle is activates when we draw our legs out to the sides. It is also in a constant state of tension to stabilize the hips.

Quadratus Lumborum

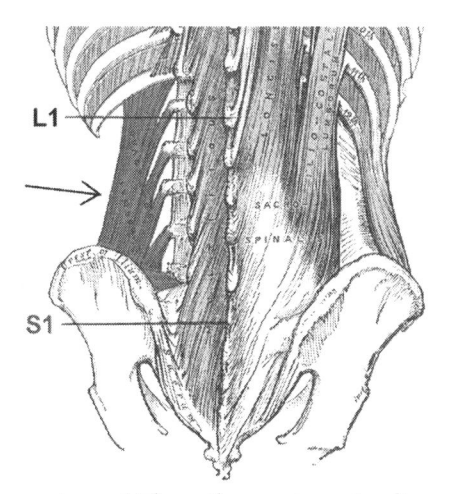

The quadratus lumborum is a deep muscle in the lower back area that originates on the iliac crest and attaches to the lumber spine and lower rib.

This muscle is one of the deep core muscles that help us to sit and stand erect. Often it is weak or not used properly because of poor posture. When the posture is aligned, this muscle will step up to the challenge of holding you upright in an efficient manner.

When used correctly, it gets very strong and can help us to sit on the floor or in meditation comfortably for a long period of time.

Asanas (Postures) for Autumn

The main aim with the autumn asana practices is to open the side of the rib cage by extending the arms overhead, activating the shoulders, strengthening the legs and stimulating the diaphragm.

Below are some asana's that achieve this aim. Incorporate these postures into your asana practice during autumn to target the lung and large intestine.

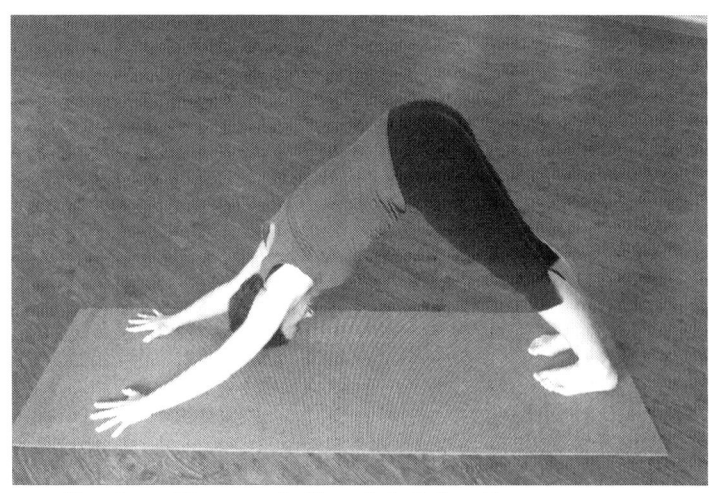

Down Facing Dog – Adho Mukha Svanasana
Main benefit – Strengthens the arms, shoulders and opens the back of legs.

1. Come onto all fours with hands underneath the shoulders and knees under the hips. Spread your fingers wide.

2. Tuck the toes under, start to extend the arms and start bringing the knees off the floor.
3. Come to extend the arms, and start to work the kegs straight. Try to bring the weight back into your legs and not so much into your arms.
4. Look to the floor just under your belly button.

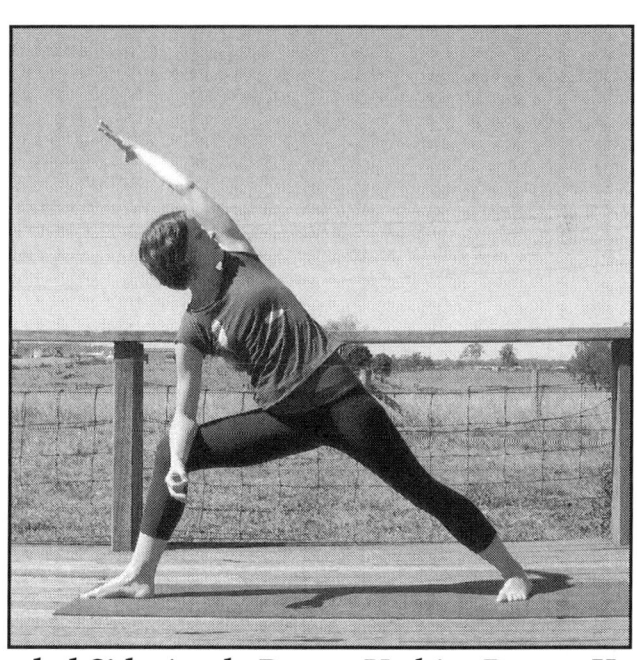

Extended Side Angle Pose – Utthita Parsva Konasana
Main Benefit – Strengthens the legs, opens the lungs and the side of the body.

1. Extend the legs wide apart and bring your right toe to face down the mat and the back toes to turn out to the side at around 45 degrees.
2. Bring your hands to your hips to start with and start to bend into the front right knee. Make sure your knee is either above your ankle or just behind it, don't let it pass over the ankle as this puts to much stress on the knee joint.

3. Bring your arms up to shoulder height, shoulders relaxed, palms facing down.
4. Now start to reach forward with your right arm, bring your torso forward also, and then place the right elbow onto the knee. Bring the left arms past your ear palm facing down. Look out to the side or up under the arm.
5. Keep your legs strong, draw the belly in, try and relax the upper body.
6. Come out by drawing the arms and torso back to centre, and releasing the legs.
7. Repeat on other side

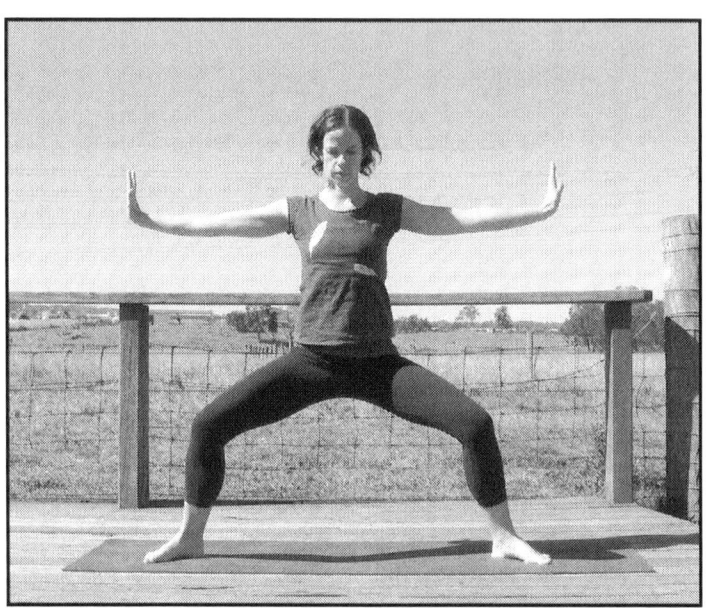

Horse Stance – Arms pushing Qi out to the side

Main Benefit – Strengthens the legs and opens the channels in the arms.

1. Bring your legs comfortable apart, feet at 45 degrees and start to sink into the knees a little. Get the sense that the knees are working outwards and work big toes into the floor.

2. Allow the tailbone to gently move towards the floor yet a low a gentle lower back curve. Basically no jamming into the lower back. Draw the anus in slightly and get a sense that the lower belly is drawn in slightly – you want to feel strong in your lower body, like a tree.
3. The arms, the branches gently push out to the sides, shoulders and elbows soft so the energy can flow easily.
4. Eyes forward, relaxed face. Close down the eyes and breath and hold for a few minutes.
5. Keep lower body strong and upper body light – you will feel the Qi intensify after a minute or two.

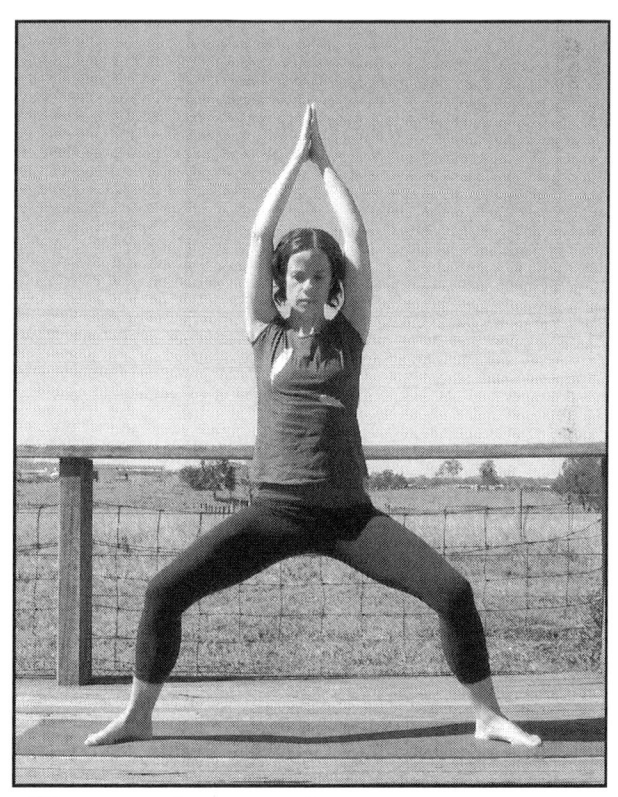

Horse Stance – Arms up in prayer
Main benefit – Strengthens the legs and stimulates Qi around the body.

1. Same stance as before, with feet out at 45 degrees and sinking comfortably into legs.
2. This time raise arms up into prayer, relaxed shoulder and elbows.
3. Breath and hold for a few minutes until string Qi sensation is felt.
4. To come out let the palms face downwards and gently let the arms downwards towards the lower belly while gently straightening the legs.

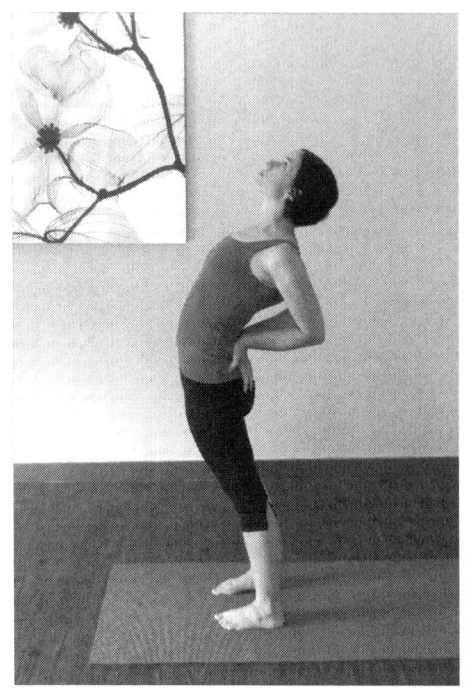

Standing Back Bend
Main Benefit –Strengthens the back of body and opens the front.

1. Place your hands, onto the lower back with finger pointing downwards.

2. Draw the elbows towards each other, such the belly in before gently drifting the hips forward and leaning back.
3. Feel the heart and throat open. Only hold for a breath then come out.
4. Come out by drawing your torso forward and releasing the arms. Feel free to move the hips around in circles to release and then try again.

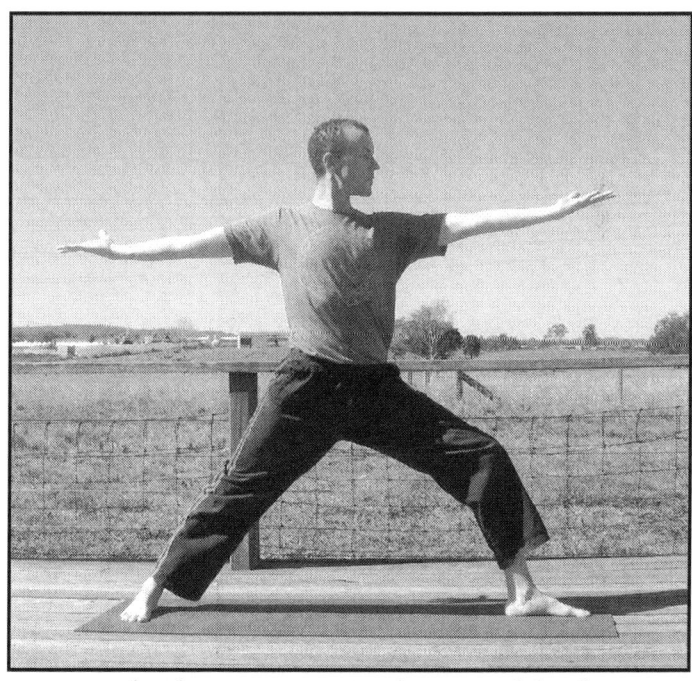

Warrior 2 (palms up version) – Virabhadrasana 2
Main benefit – Strengthens the legs and opens the arm channels.

1. Bring your legs wide apart. Turn your left toes to the front of the mat and your back toes around 45 degrees.
2. Bring your hands onto your hips to start with and sink into your left knee, making sure that the left knee remains either above or just behind the ankle joint.
3. Get solid in the legs, tuck the belly in slightly

4. Then extend the arms out at shoulder height and turn the palms upwards. Soften the shoulder and the elbows so that the Qi can move easily.
5. Gazing down the front arm –extending your Qi through your eyes.
6. Spread the fingers wide to encourage the Qi to move into the hands.
7. You can pull the finger back towards the body to emphasis the Qi in the wrists and hands, and then draw the finger up the other way to open the other side of the wrist.
8. Stay for a few minutes with a steady breath until you can feel the Qi intensify.
9. To come out release the arms and straighten out the legs and release.
10. Repeat on the other side.

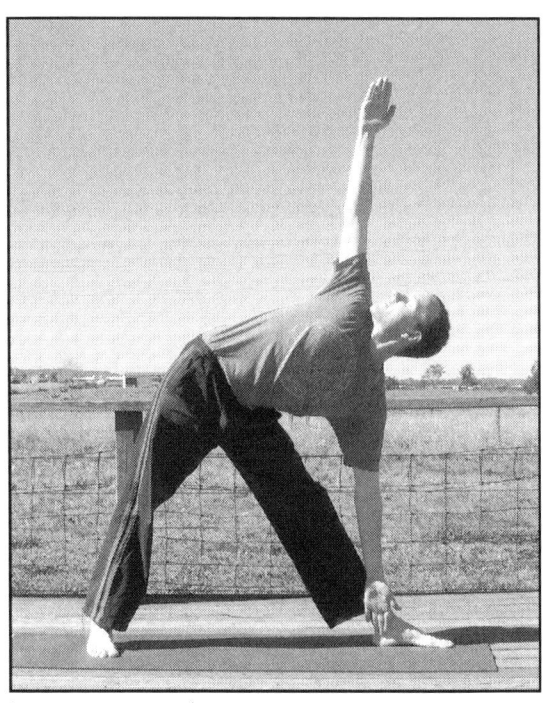

Triangle Pose - Trikonasana

Main Benefit – Opens the side of the body.

1. Bring your feet to about 1 meter apart (not as wide as the warrior 2 pose).
2. Turn the left toes to face the front of the mat and the back toes about 45 to 90 degrees.
3. Bring both arms up to shoulder height, keep your legs straight and then start to bring your arms and torso to the front of the mat as far as you can go.
4. Then simply draw your left arm down onto the left leg, above the ankle a few inches and draw the right arm up to the sky.
5. Keep the chest open. Look to the floor, out to the side or, if the neck is ok try tucking the chin into the right shoulder and look up towards top hand.
6. Keep your legs active by pulling up on the kneecaps. Keep the belly sucked in slightly, steady breathing.
7. Get a sense of pushing the right hip out to the side.
8. Hold for a few breaths and when ready, come out by softening the knees and drawing yourself up.
9. Repeat on the other side.

Yoga for the Seasons

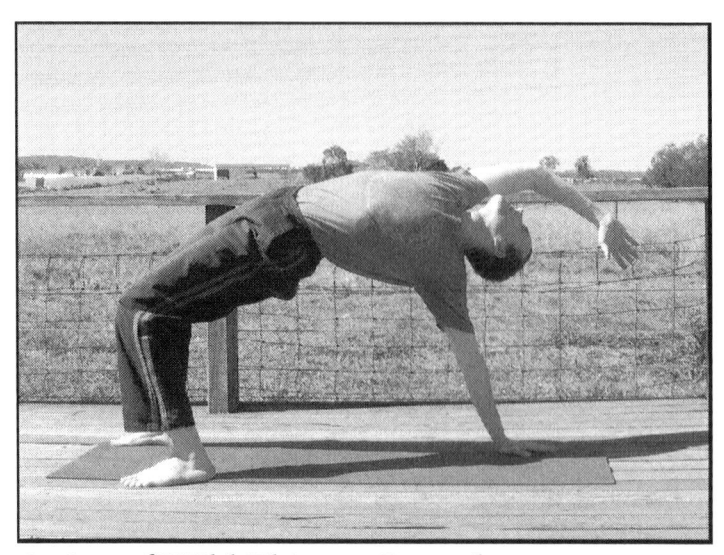

Variation of Wild Thing – Camatkarasana

Main Benefit – Opens the front of the torso, belly, lungs and chest.

Caution - This is an intermediate to advanced pose so only attempt it if you have been doing yoga for some time already.

1. Start in down facing dog.
2. Gently bend the knees and place your left foot underneath you and over the right side about 20cm or so to the side of your other foot.
3. Then keeping the knees bent slightly, allow the feet to pivot and draw the right arm off the floor to roll over into the backbend.
4. Extend the right arm behind you, and keep your hips working upwards.
5. Only hold for a breath or two and then to come out draw the right arm back in, pivot on the feet and then place the left foot back into the down facing dog position also placing the right hand back into down dog position.
6. Repeat to the other side.

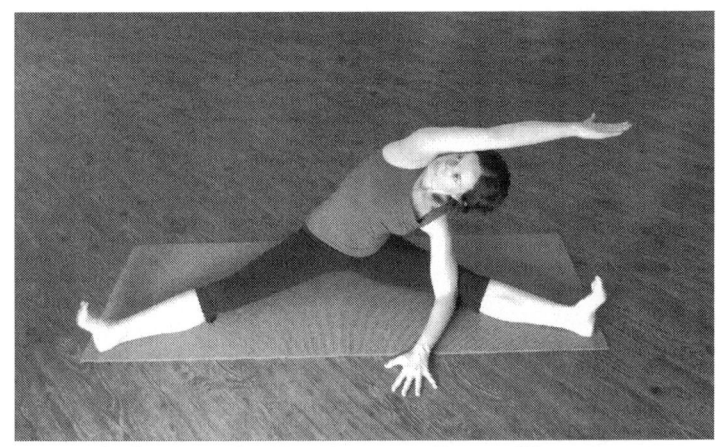

Sitting Side Bend - Parivrttta Janu Sirsasana
Main Benefit – Opens the side of the lungs and torso.

1. Bring the left leg straight out to about 45 degrees and the right knee bent with right foot into inner left thigh.
2. Then bring both arms up above the head, draw the belly in and then start to drift the arms and torso over to left leg slightly twisting the torso.
3. Bring the left arm down to the left eg, or floor, wherever it works for you and continue to let the top right arm drift towards the left leg.
4. You can look out to the side or if the neck is ok and you can keep your chest open, try looking up underneath the top arm.
5. Keep your belly slightly drawn in with this pose.
6. Use your exhalation breath to soften into the pose and the inhalation breath to lengthen.
7. Stay for at least a few good, deep breaths, close your eyes if you like.
8. To come out simply draw your torso back towards centre and rest the arms.
9. Repeat to the other side

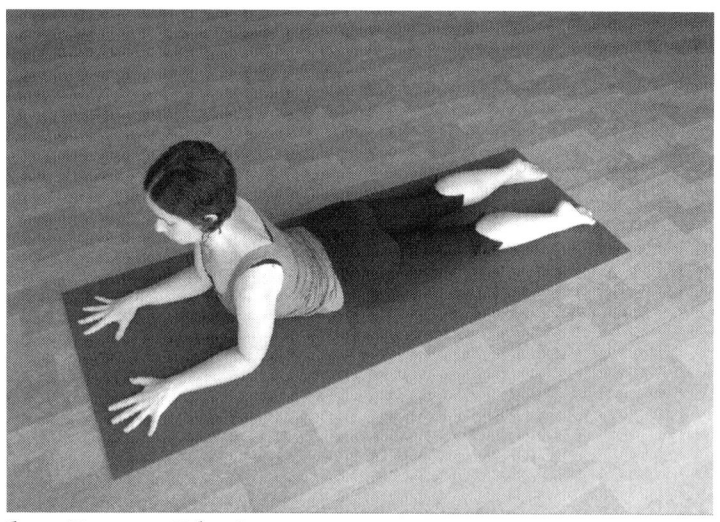

Cobra Pose – Bhujangasana

Main Benefit – A gentle back bend that promotes a healthy lower back arch.

1. Start by lying on your belly on your mat. Feet hip width apart, tops of the fleet flat.
2. Arms just underneath the shoulder or just in front of shoulders.
3. Start pushing the hips gently into the floor and raising the chest and head of the floor without any support from hands.
4. Then start to add the extra support from the hands to help you raise the torso up to where it works for you. It's different for everybody so listen to your body and don't aim to do the same height as you see in pictures or videos. You don't have to have your arms straight – the back is the most important, listen to that!
5. Only stay up for a breath and then come back down onto your belly.
6. This pose is good to repeat throughout the class.
7. At the beginning of a class or routine only come up a little, when the body is warmed up then you can go a bit higher.

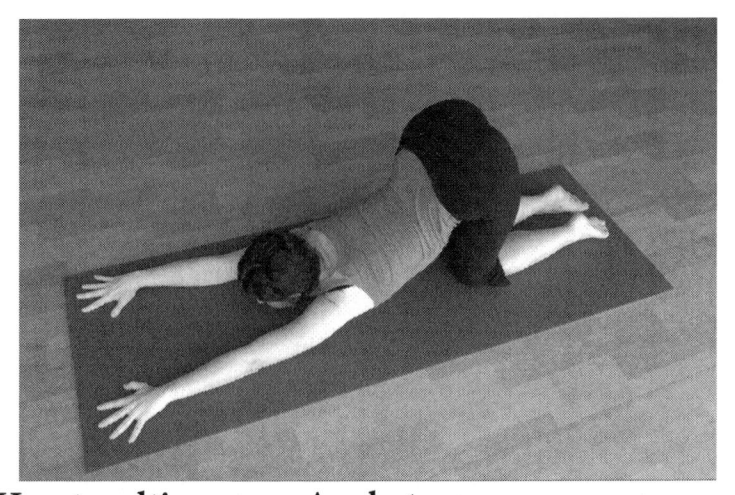

Heart melting pose- Anahatasana
Main Benefit – Opens the heart, lungs and shoulders.

1. Start on all fours, hands below the shoulders and knees under the hips. Tops of the feet flat.
2. Keep your buttocks above your knees and start to walk your hands out in front and allow your heart to sink towards the floor.
3. Rest your head wherever is comfortable, on the chin, forehead or on side of face.
4. Allow the back to relax and the shoulders to open.
5. Stay for a minute or two and then to come up simply walk your hands back up into all fours.

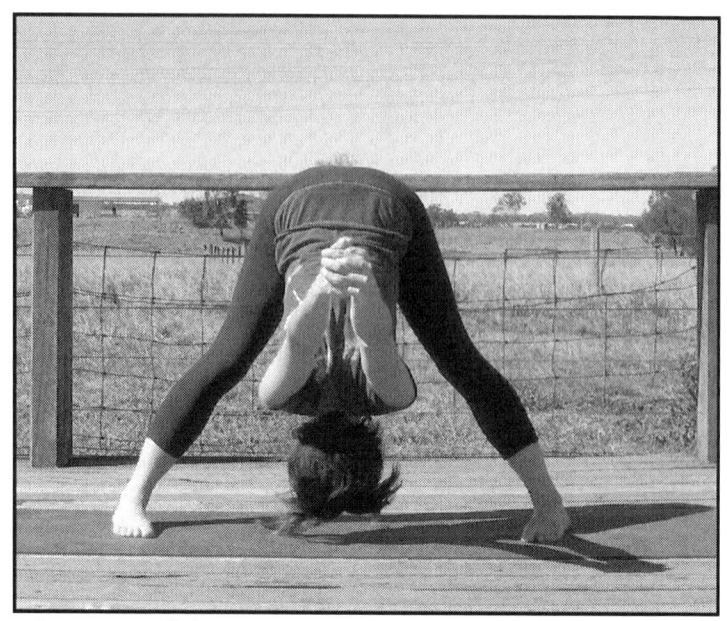

Wide Legged forward Bend (variation) – Prasarita Padottanasana

Main Benefit – Opens the channels in the arms and the Shoulders.

1. Take a wide legged stance with toes both facing to the side of the room.
2. Interlace your hands behind your back while upright. Then inhale, lengthen your spine upwards and then as you exhale start to stick your buttocks out behind and draw the torso forward and down while letting the arms drift up behind you.
3. Allow a few breaths to settle into this pose – keep breathing and relax your head.
4. When you're ready to come up, bend your knees slightly, and imagine someone is behind you pulling you up by your arms bringing you upright.
5. Relax the arms and release the legs.

Other techniques that stimulate the Lungs and Large Intestine:

Lion's Breath

1. Come to sit in a comfortable position with a straight spine (Seiza if comfortable)
2. Take a deep breath in through the nose and lean back slightly.
3. As you begin to exhale, start to bring your torso forward. Open your mouth, stick out your tongue, open your eyes as wide as possible, and breath out through your mouth as you drift your torso forward. Empty out the lungs.
4. Relax the face and repeat about 3 times.

Self massage of the Internal Organs

1. Start by gently working the fingers into the abdominal cavity, just below the belly button. Then work your way up the right hands side of the abdominal cavity moving slowly.
2. Move around the belly area like a face of a clock returning back to below the belly button.
3. Then relax and have some water. It can make you feel a bit weird for a while afterwards to just sit down or rest and let things return to 'normal'.

Tapping the Arms and Chest Area with Loose Fists (a Qi Gong technique)

1. Use one hand at a time to gently pummel the opposite side of the chest.
2. Then slowly move the pummel down the inside of the opposite arm. When you reach the ringer, turn the arm over and pummel up the outside of the arm back up to the shoulder and over to the lungs.
3. Repeat 3 rounds on each side.

Metal Element Daily Lifestyle Practices

- Early morning walks to bring fresh Qi energy into the lungs.

- Cover / protect your neck area from the wind.

- Refine your character – identify what qualities you wish to cultivate in yourself and let go of anything that may be holding you back from that, e.g. memories, opinions, people, places, fears, worries etc.

- Breath awareness meditation / present moment awareness cultivation.

- Metal is about structure so re-affirm structure in your life. Be consistent and focus on the long-term goals over the short-term highs - Be disciplined but not rigid.

- Tie up loose ends and then let them go.

- Start withdrawing from excessive activity or over committing yourself.

- Strip away the non-essentials. Refine and articulate.

- Go to bed a little earlier than usual. Always best to get to bed before 11pm.

Supporting the Other Elements to Assist the Metal Element

As outlined in the 5 elements Chapter, if we want to balance out the metal element we also need to take into consideration the elements that feed the Metal Element. This is especially in the case of any illness or disease related to the lungs or large intestine. The elements that nourish and support the Metal element are the Earth element (*Shen* cycle) and the Wood element (*Ko* cycle).

Earth Element Nourishment

- Warm foods with a little spice
- Avoid damp cold foods and drinks
- Take your time to eat a nourishing breakfast (eg. porridge)
- Eat slowly
- Weights, resistance training (morning is best).

Wood Element Stimulation and Harmonization

- Increase any movement-based activities, dance more, try a new movement class and commit to a more regular yoga asana practice. (Liver energy loves to move)
- Moderate and reduce coffee, alcohol and spicy foods
- Launch new projects, get inspired and be more social

Food / Oriental Diet Therapy ~
Autumn

For autumn the following foods and methods are recommended in nourishing and supporting all of the organs at this time of year.

Grains: Brown rice, white rice, oats

Vegetables: Brussels sprouts, Asparagus, Broccoli, Celery, cauliflower, cabbage, Chinese cabbage, celery, daikon radish, onions, parsnips, watercress, mustard and turnip greens, turnips, garlic, cucumber, leeks

Beans and Pulses: Navy, Soy

Fruits: Banana, pear, apples

Fish: Bass, snapper, cod, haddock, herring, flounder, sole, halibut

Herbs and Seasonings: dill, fennel, thyme, ginger root, horseradish, cinnamon, cayenne, basil, and rosemary

Avoid / Reduce
- Salads
- Too many raw foods
- Cold drinks
- Dairy
- Oily damp foods
- Alcohol

Oriental Yoga

- White sugar
- White flour

Herbs to Support Lungs and Large Intestine

Here is a list of herbs that support the main organs involved in the keeping the lungs and large intestine healthy. Again, taking herbs alongside a healthy lifestyle that incorporates yoga will provide more effective results. Just taking herbs without engaging in other supportive methods will often bring little results.

Herbs that stimulate the digestion and help flush the intestines will help keep the large intestine from becoming stagnant and toxic. Please seek guidance from a health professional (naturopath, Herbalist, Chinese herbalist, Chinese medicine practitioner) for more information about correct dosages or for treating specific conditions.

Astragalus – Increases lung Qi and supports immune system

Vitamin C – More of a vitamin than a herb but worth mentioning. It's cheap and effective. Cleans out the liver and organs, repairs tissue, natural anti-depressant and supports the immune system, just to name a few. Around 3 grams a day is a suitable dose, however please seek advice from a health practitioner on dosages if experiencing any adverse effects.

Liquorice – Stimulates digestion and acts as an anti-inflammatory

Dandelion Root - Detoxes the liver (wood element), stimulates digestion

Ginseng - Tones spleen and stomach (earth element) and nourishes the kidneys. Also acts as a healthy energy tonic.

Green Tea - Tones stomach and spleen (earth element), digestive stimulant, clears mind

Cinnamon - Stimulates digestion and supports fire element

Autumn Meditations

Taoist Lung Energy Meditation

Preparation: Sit in a comfortable position. If you are sitting on the floor I always recommend sitting up on a folded blanket - ideally you want your knees to be just below your hips. This will help you sit for longer periods without extra stress in your back. When you're comfortably seated, place your hands in a comfortable position. I generally recommend interlacing the fingers and placing them on your lap or just in front of your lap, or simply place one palm on top of the other. When you place the hands this way it generates a very nurturing energy and helps one draw the energy inwards for regeneration. You can of course place the hands on the knees. This position, I find, tends to be more suited to an opening and expanding type of energy, good for sending out energy and metta (loving kindness).

Ok, so then close down the eyes and settle into a relaxed posture. Find your breath moving through the nostrils and keep watching it. Just have your attention on your breath, let any thoughts just move through your mind without giving them any attention. Relinquish the mind's thoughts and images as they arise. Come back to the breath with an alert yet relaxed awareness. Just watch the breath for at least five minutes until the mind starts to settle.

So when the mind has settled a little, move your awareness down to your lungs and your chest cavity. As you breath feel the breath fill the lungs and you can simply say something like this to your lungs, "thank you lungs, thank you for helping me to breath. I love and appreciate you and your hard work." The intention is generate and cultivate appreciation and gratitude towards your lungs.

You can visualize a white, grey cloud being drawn into the lungs and swirling around the chest cavity allowing it to dissolve any blockages or impurities. Also set the intention for it to dissolve any excess grief or sadness that may be stored there. Be sure to keep a deep exhalation breath going while doing this meditation.

After a few minutes, draw your attention to the front of the throat. Feel the breath enter through the front of the throat, cooling and nourishing your lungs as it travels through the throat and into the lungs. You can add an internal mantra to the breath. So as you breath in, focus your attention on the throat and say to yourself "Hummmmm" and as you breathe out, say to yourself "Saaaaaaaa".

Do this for a few minutes.

After some time, begin to visualize a gentle smile in the area of the lungs and chest area. Send the smile down to your chest, your heart, lungs and throat. Give thanks by smiling to them and then see them smiling back at you.

To complete bring your attention back to the breath at the nostrils. Let go of all other practices. Watch the breath until you feel calm and relaxed. Then when ready, open the eyes gently and release your posture.

Letting Go Meditation

This one is very simple to explain, yet often difficult to practice. You can do this while in a formal meditation posture or you can do it anywhere really – any situation that doesn't require you to think, which is probably about 80% of the time.

As you sit, after eating a meal, on a park bench, while waiting for the bus, while doing a yoga pose, walking on the beach or even driving, just relinquish thoughts as they arise. Your mind has a habit of always throwing words and images into your head but you don't have to follow them or give them any importance. Instead, just don't follow them, let them pass through. If you find your breath and just watch yourself breathing, this can give you an anchor to focus on. Again, when images and thoughts arise, don't give them any importance. Allow the space to come in. Allow the space rather than cultivating thoughts and stories in the mind.

See if you can sit for at least five minutes while doing this. And practice doing it more and more often.

Life has a magical way of just doing its thing and working things out in its own way, so you don't need to really think or stress out about much of it at all. Most thought simply serves as a distraction to the present moment that is life. When we are in thinking mode, we are missing the moment. It's the same with emotions. If anger arises, watch it, don't follow it, don't give it any importance. The same goes for any thoughts attached to it. Let it pass—let it go. If you keep practicing this, the emotions and the habit of excess thinking lose their intensity and power, and your life will automatically settle into a much more stable and peaceful place. You don't have to force anything to happen - just let go of the excess thoughts and unhelpful emotions and the rest will take care of itself.

It is really that simple! Let go of the grudges, let go of the drama, let go of the self-righteousness, let go of your anger and you will have more access to the present moment, to life.

Water Element

~ Winter ~

Kidney and Bladder

Water element is next. Let's have a look at the 5-elements to see where the Water element sits within the cosmic dance.

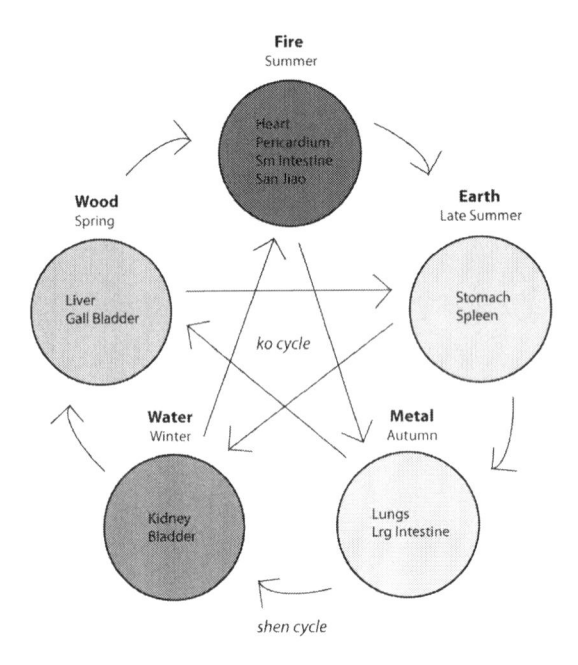

Figure 1.3

When we look at figure 1.3, we can see that the Water element is supported by the Metal element in the *Shen* (nurturing) cycle and the Earth element supports Water in the *Ko (controlling)* cycle. I will talk a little more about the Metal element and Wood element later on in this book.

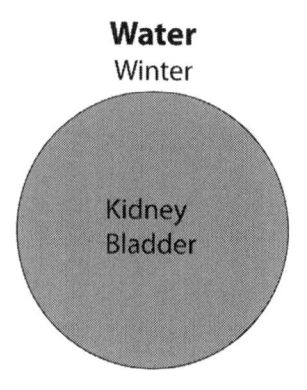

Water
Winter

Kidney
Bladder

Winter (Water element) is the most 'yin' time of the year. Meaning it's the best time to withdraw from excessive activity, to sleep more, eat more, slow down and spend more time in self-enquiry. The organs associated with winter are the kidneys and the bladder. The kidneys, in Oriental medicine, are one of the most important organs and energies of our system for the kidneys store the vital energy, known as Jing Qi. Jing Qi is our most potent essence of energy that trickles out throughout our lifetime to bring us a long life. Basically, when we run out of Jing Qi, we pass away because this vital life energy to sustain our bodies has run out. We can easily and prematurely use up this Jing Qi through excessive activity, excessive stress, worry, drugs, alcohol, stimulants, addictive behaviors and by generally not taking enough time out to relax and regenerate. This is what the winter energy is all about - to take time out to replenish and regenerate so that when the other seasons come around, we have a healthy source of energy to work with. Adrenal fatigue and chronic fatigue are common occurrence in our western fast-paced society, and these conditions are signs that we have taxed the kidney's energies too much and have not taken enough time out to relax and regenerate. If we keep running ourselves into the ground, we will end up very miserable, depleted, fatigued and likely to die at an earlier age. Deep, achy pains in the lower back, poor bone health (weak bones, tooth decay), hearing loss, weak knees and fatigue are all signs that the kidneys are depleted and need some love.

The kidneys and bladder are all about <u>nourishment</u> and <u>replenishment</u> on all levels.

Water Organ Physiology

Let's have a look at these Kidney and Bladder and how they function according to Western medicine and Oriental medicine.

Kidney function (Western Medicine)

- Removes waste from blood
- Regulates salts and acids (pH levels)
- Produces hormones that help control blood pressure, water balance, make red blood cells and maintain strong bones

Bladder Function (Western Medicine)

- Storage of urine
- The release of urine by its own muscle system

Kidney Function (Oriental Medicine)

- Storing essence (Jing Qi) given at birth
- Dominates human reproduction and development
- Produces 'marrow' to fill the brain
- Produces 'marrow' for bone health
- Manufactures blood
- Manifests in hair on the head
- Opens into the ears
- Fluid secretions mainly urine, semen and vaginal fluids
- Houses will-power, courage, inner strength
- Emotions associated are anxiety, fear and courage

Bladder Function (Oriental Medicine)

- Fluid transformation
- Stores and excretes urine

Physical, Emotional & Spiritual Signs and Symptoms (Oriental medicine)

Kidney & Bladder <u>In Balance</u>

- Have courage, inner strength and will-power
- Ability to be calm, clear and grounded (can handle stress better than most, doesn't get too stressed out and knows when its time to pull back and reduce activity)
- Patient and persistent
- Thick head of hair and good hearing
- Likely to have high brain function and the potential for highly developed intelligence
- Fertile, can reproduce easily and produce healthy, well-developed children
- Healthy, balanced sexual life (not too much, not too little)
- Strong and stable back body
- Strong bones and a sense of solidity in the body frame
- A powerful charismatic presence
- Able to fall asleep easily and have healthy, deep and regular sleep
- Meditation and relaxation come without much effort

Kidney and Bladder <u>Out Of Balance</u>

- Easily startled, jumpy, fearful, anxious, agitated, restless
- Lower back pains or deep achy back pain
- Very tired, very lethargic

- Lacks courage and inner strength to launch new projects or pursue new avenues (work, career, travel, etc)
- Lacks inner fire, passion, motivation and luster
- Ungrounded – sometimes quick to neurotic behavior and anger
- Pale face
- Very low sex drive or excessive sex drive
- Infertile or very hard to reproduce
- Urinates very frequently with clear urine, painful urination or urinary incontinence
- Carries excess fluids
- Poor short-term memory
- Fickle, unsteady mind
- Ringing in the ears, hearing loss
- Osteoporosis, bone weaknesses, tooth decay
- Impaired mental development
- Thin hair
- Hot flashes
- Dry mouth and skin
- Prone to kidney and bladder infections

The main causes responsible for draining the kidney and bladder are stress, succumbing to and re-affirming fear-based behavior and excess activity like overworking or excess physical training. One's genes and bodily constitution also play a role in the overall health of the kidney's energy. Therefore, if one knows their bodily constitution is not ideal, then extra caution is advised to not overwork and drain the kidney's energy. Instead, devoting to a slower and more nurturing lifestyle is advisable as it helps build up the kidney energies over time.

The Water Element Meridians

Winter is directly associated with the kidney and bladder organs and meridians, so let's take a closer look at these meridians and where they travel.

Kidney Meridian

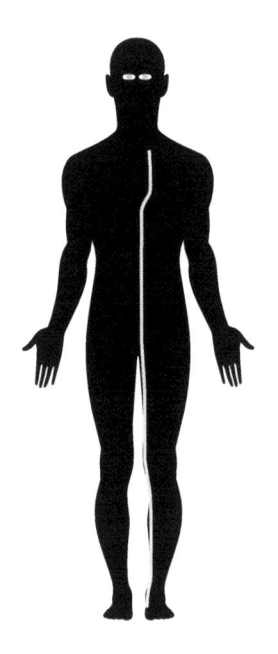

This channel includes the lowest acupuncture point on the body. Starting on the sole of the foot, it rises up the inside of the foot and loops around the inner ankle. It then begins to rise up the inner leg and up to the groin where it goes internal and connects up with the base of the spine, the kidneys and the bladder. It re-emerges at the pubic area and then travels up the front of the body, over the abdomen and finishes just under the collarbone. There are also many other internal channels going on that connect up most of the organs in the body. The multitude of internal channels help to deliver the Jing Qi and deeper internal energies to nurture all the organs, therefore, making it one of the most important and crucial meridians and organs.

Bladder Meridian

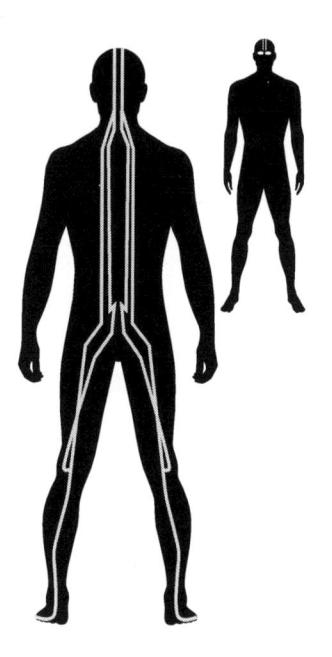

The bladder channel is the longest channel in the body. It begins at the inner corner of the eye and rises up over the top of the head where it goes into the brain. It re-emerges at the back of the head, and as it begins to descend down onto the back, it divides into two branches that both run parallel with the spine. At the area of the lumbar region, an internal branch connects to the kidneys and the bladder and then re-emerges to travel down the buttocks to the back of the knee. The outer branch travels all the way down, over the buttocks and down the centre of the back of the legs. This newly single channel passes behind the outer ankle and travels to the tip of the little toe.

Muscles Associated with the Kidneys

The following are the muscles that are associated with the kidney meridian.

Psoas muscle

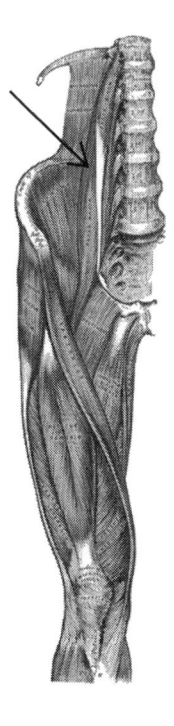

The psoas muscle is a deep muscle in the hip area. It originates at the transverse process of the lumber spine and travels inside the pelvis and attaches to the lesser trochanter of the femur (thigh bone).

The psoas is one of the most important muscles to do with the lower back, the hips and sitting posture, in general. Often, the psoas muscle is too contracted, due to sitting in chairs or driving for too many hours of the day, day in day out, causing the psoas muscle to be shortened. Signs of a shortened psoas muscle are a rounded lower back, difficulty in standing up straight, tail bone tucked under and weak abdominal muscles - which all are contributing factors to back pain.

Iliacus

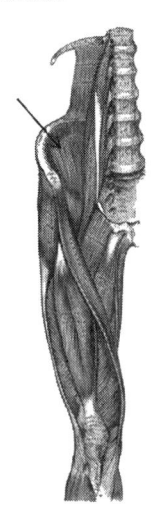

The iliacus originates from the iliac fossa, on the interior side of the hipbone. It joins forces with the psoas muscle, running down the inside of the hipbone and attaches to the lesser trochanter.

The Upper Trapezius

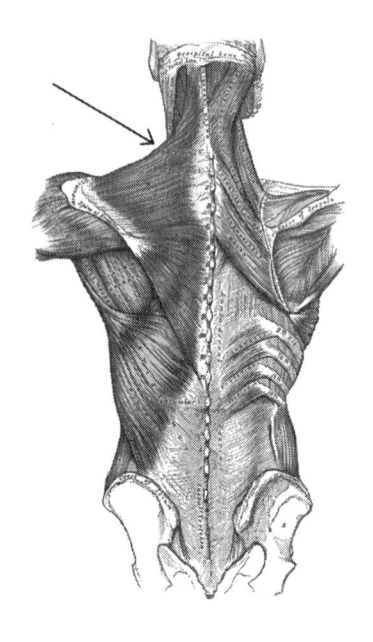

The trapezius is a large superficial muscle that travels from the occipital bone to the lower thoracic vertebrae. The trapezius is divided into three sections, the upper, the middle and the lower, all of which have slightly different tasks.

The upper trapezius is what we are to focus on here. It originates from the base of the skull (the occipital bones) where they proceed downward and outward where they attach onto the posterior border of the clavicle (collarbone). Its main task is to simply support the weight of the arms as they attach to the neck and head.

Nearly everyone has a tight and stressed trapezius muscle. I have probably only meet two or three people in my life in which this muscle was not in some kind of stress. You can easily notice it in people, as their shoulders are quite high and their neck space is not very open or free. Often it's associated with fear. It's a type of defensive mechanism where the body has gone into protective mode. It also indicates that they tend to be very anxious about the future and therefore, don't carry much faith or ease with life – they tend to take on all the responsibility of life, feeling as though they are in control or need to maintain control. Help to get out of this unhelpful pattern comes by simply moving your awareness into your shoulders at least a few times a day. As you discover the tension, allow yourself to let go, release and relax. The universe is working with you and for you!

Awareness is the key to releasing tension and changing the behavior of these muscles – you can get a massage therapist to pummel it for hours and get it to release, but if you don't add awareness to the process, the muscles will quickly go back into the old behavior pattern. Become aware of what triggers you to bring tension into your shoulders. When you identify what triggers the behavior, and are in that situation, keep your awareness in the shoulders and keep telling your brain to let it go. It takes a bit of effort, but after some time, its intensity dissipates and a new behavior will be formed. If you aren't aware of your behavior, how can you expect it to change? And just to clarify, it's not somebody else or some external situation that is the cause of your tension, it's your reaction and your response to the situation that causes the tension inside.

Muscles Associated with the Bladder

The following are the muscles that are associated with the bladder meridian.

Erector Spinae Muscles (Sacrospinalis)

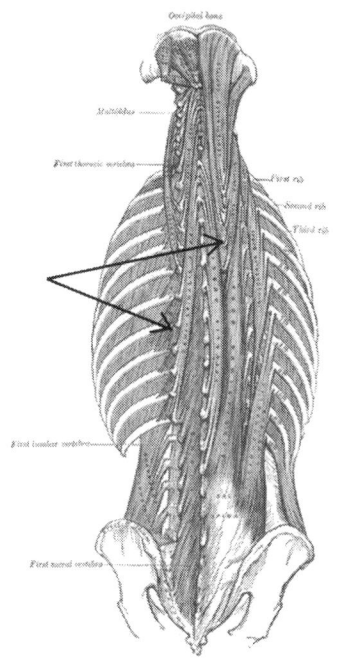

The erector spinae muscle is not just one muscles but a bundle of deep muscles and tendons that run up either side of the spine. The mass and combined strength of these muscles and tendons differ at different parts of the vertebral column. They are a great example of the amazing complexity and interconnectedness of the human musculoskeletal system.

These muscles are mainly involved in keeping the vertebral column upright in a balanced and efficient manner. In most cases, these muscles are weakened and over flexed by the rounded back posture created from sitting in poorly designed furniture or from the rounding of our backs when sitting at computer desks and playing with little digital devices.

Posterior Tibialis

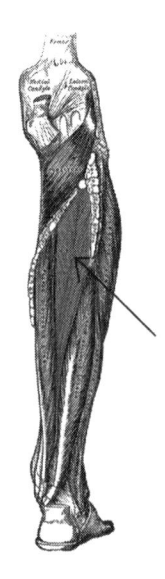

The posterior tibialis is the most central of the lower leg muscles. It originates on the inner posterior borders of the fibula and tibia and runs down the leg and attaches at a variety of ankle and foot bones.

Its main job is to stabilize the lower leg. A dysfunction or weakness in these muscles often results in flat feet.

Anterior Tibial

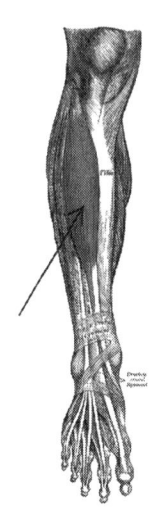

The anterior tibialis muscle is a superficial muscle located at the font of the lower leg. It originates at the upper lateral part of the tibia and inserts into the cuneiform and first metatarsal bone of the foot.

Its main job is to dosiflex (pull toes back) and invert the foot. This muscle is usually quite tender to massage. It's a good place to massage if you're looking to rejuvenate your legs from walking and you are looking for more energy.

Peroneus

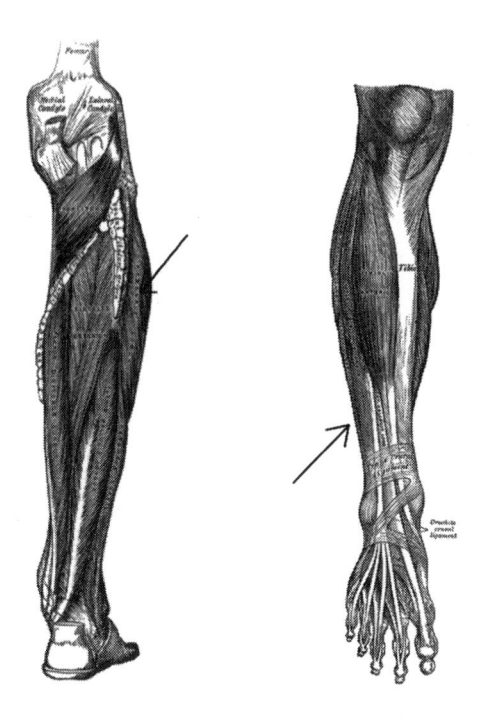

The peroneus muscles are a group of three superficial muscles, (longus, brevis and tertius) that all originate on the fibula and insert onto the metatarsals in the foot. Their main job is to dorsiflex (toes pulled back) or planter flex (toes pointing away) the foot and externally rotate the foot.

Asanas (Postures) for Winter

The main aim with the winter asana practices is to open the bladder channel on the back, strengthen and tone the muscles in the back of the body and tone the deep muscles in the hips. Below are some asanas that achieve this aim.

Incorporate these postures into your asana practice during winter to stimulate and nourish the kidneys and the bladder.

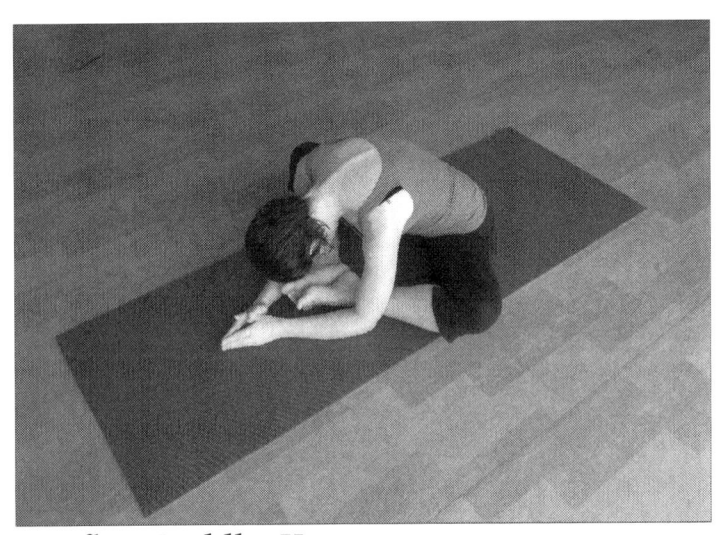

Butterfly – Buddha Konasana
Main benefit – Opens the inner legs and opens the back of the body.

Oriental Yoga

1. Sitting on the floor or up on some folded blankets, bring the soles of your feet together. Give yourself some space between your groin and your feet.
2. Grabbing hold of your feet, inhale to lengthen the spine, exhale to draw your heart space down toward your feet and the floor.
3. Allow yourself to move into this pose slowly. While deep in the pose, really focus on relaxing your legs and knees toward the floor. Relax your back and draw your head toward the floor, relaxing the back of your neck and shoulder. Close your eyes and breathe here for a few minutes.
4. When you're ready to come up, simply roll up slowly back into a sitting position with your back straight.

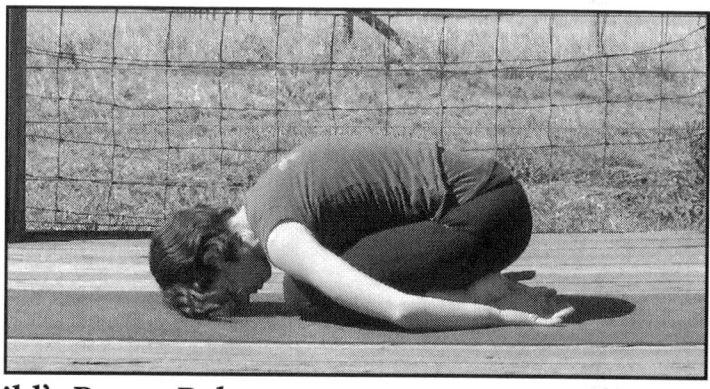

Child's Pose – Balasana

Main benefit – Calms the mind, draws energy inside and softens the back.

1. Sit on your heels, feet flat in the seiza position. If it's too much on your ankles or knees, try placing a blanket under your feet and knees. If this doesn't work for you, then just come down into a cross-legged seated position.
2. From here, simply draw your torso down toward the floor. Rest your forehead on the floor. Relaxed arms can be out in front or down the side.

3. Close your eyes and take a few breaths, relax your back and shoulders.
4. When you're ready to come out, simply draw your torso back up to sit on your heels or on the floor.
- The child's pose can be done anytime you feel like you need to have a rest or break, especially in yoga class.

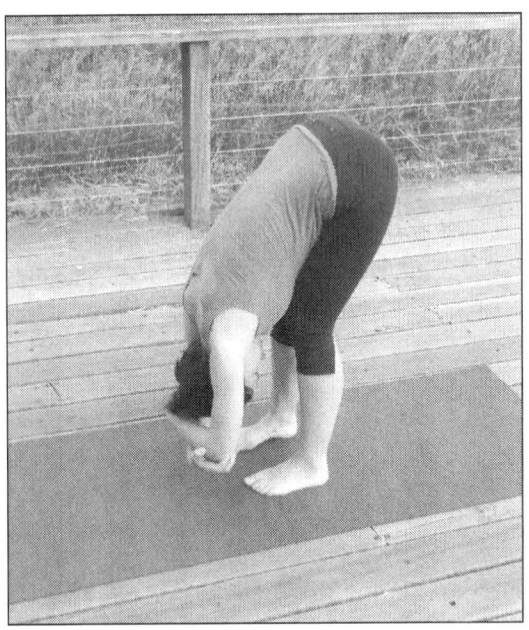

Forward Bend – Uttanasana
Main benefit – Opens the back of the body and draws energy inside.

1. Bring both feet hip width apart at the front of the mat.
2. As you inhale, bring both hands above your head as you stand to lengthen yourself out, then as you exhale, soften your arms, bend your knees and draw your torso down toward the floor into the forward bend.
3. Make sure your knees are a little bent, so you can focus on relaxing your head, neck and arms.
4. Stay for a few breaths, closing your eyes if you like.

5. To come up, bend into your knees, tuck your tailbone under and start to roll yourself up into a standing position.

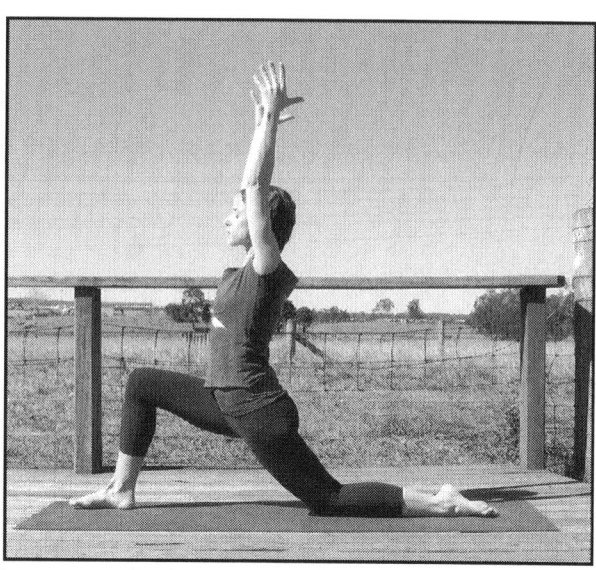

Low Lunge – Anjaneyasana

Main benefit – Opens the psoas muscle, the front of the body and strengthens the back.

1. Ideally, you will start in a standing-forward, bent position (Uttanasana) at the front of the mat. Then simply step your left leg to the back of the mat and bring your back knee to the floor, the top of your back foot should be flat on the floor.
2. Make sure your front ankle is either just in front of or directly underneath your front knee.
3. Open your heart up and bring your arms out to the side, and then bring them up above your head. In this picture, the hands are shoulder width apart – this makes it easier to relax the shoulders down away from the ears. You can bring your hands together too if that feels more natural.
4. Allow your lower back to lengthen and gently work your hips forward and down toward the floor, opening the front of your left hip.

5. After a few breaths, bring your torso and your arms down toward the floor, tuck your back toe under and step to the front of the mat, returning to your forward bend at the front of the mat.
6. Repeat on the other side.

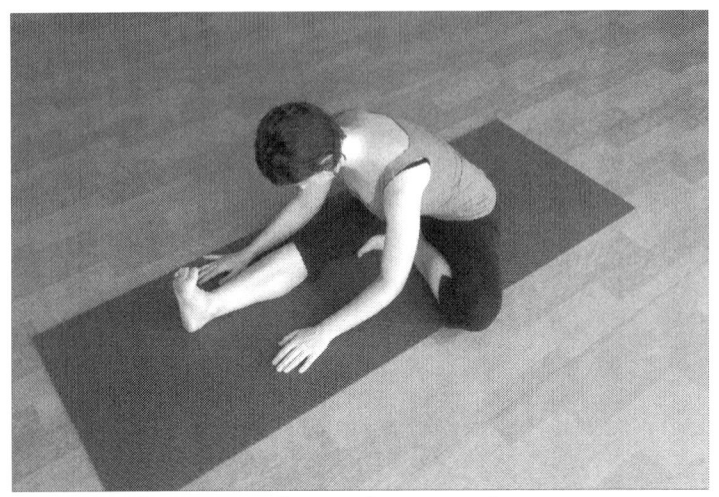

One Legged Forward Bend - Janu Sirsasana

Main benefit – Opens the back of the legs and the back of the body.

1. Sitting on the floor or up on some folded blankets, bring your left leg out in front and bend your right knee so you can place your right foot on the inside of your left leg.
2. As you inhale, raise your arms above your head and lengthen out your spine, then as you exhale, draw your arms, torso and head forward and down the midline of your body.
3. Let your arms rest wherever they are comfortable. Stay for many breaths, using your inhalation to lengthen the spine and the exhalation to soften forward and down.
4. After some time then allow your back to round as your neck and head soften toward the floor. Enjoy this different style of stretching for a few breaths.

5. To come out, slowly roll yourself back up to a sitting position with your back straight.

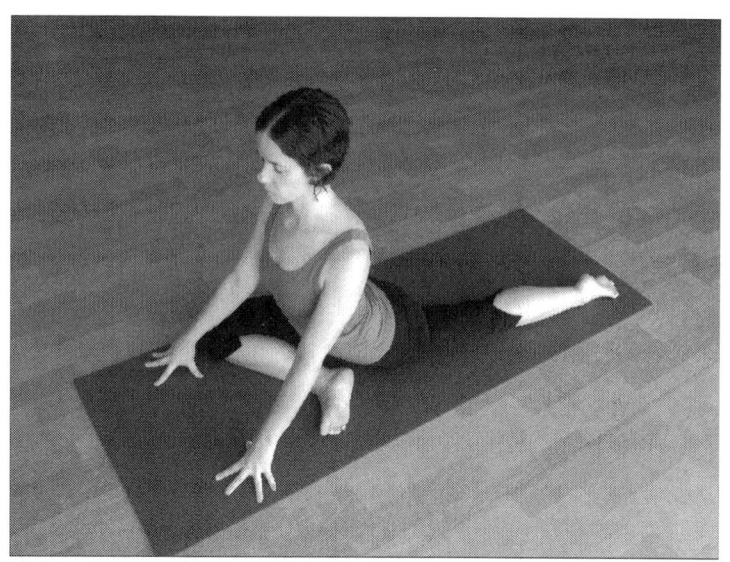

One Legged Pigeon Pose – Eka Pada Rajakapotasana
Main benefit – Opens the hips, legs and buttocks.

1. Start on all fours on the mat - knees underneath your hips and hands under your shoulders.
2. Draw your right knee up to your right wrist. Then, allow your back leg to slide out behind you so your hips come closer to the floor.
3. You can wiggle your front right foot out to the left a little to increase the stretch.
4. Make sure your hips are just off the floor and squared toward the front of the mat. You can place a blanket underneath your right buttocks for extra support, if it feels better for you.
5. As you inhale, open your heart toward the sky and as you exhale, draw your torso forward and down toward the floor. Relax your arms into any position that supports you. Find a position where you can relax your upper body, head, neck and arms.

Yoga for the Seasons

6. Take many deep breaths and allow yourself to sink deeper. Close your eyes if you like.
7. When ready to come out, bring your hands beside your head and use them to draw yourself up. Then slide your right knee back into the all fours position again. Wiggle out your legs if you need to.
8. Repeat on the other side.

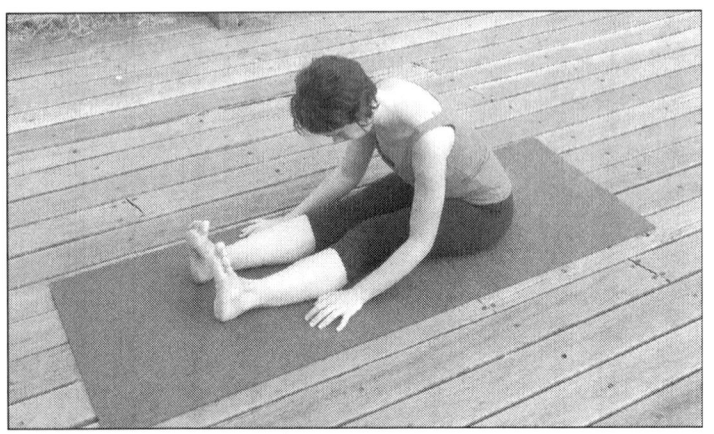

Forward Bend - Paschimottanasana
Main benefit – Opens the back of the body and draws energy inside.

1. Sit on the floor or up on some folded blankets (like I am in this picture).
2. Sitting up nice and tall, inhale to raise your arms up and create length in your spine, then as you exhale draw your arms, torso and head forward and down.
3. Take your time to get into this one. Let your arms rest wherever they may.
4. Keep focusing on releasing your head and neck toward the floor. Close your eyes if you like.
5. Hold for many breaths and when ready to come out, simply roll yourself up, back into a sitting with your spine straight.

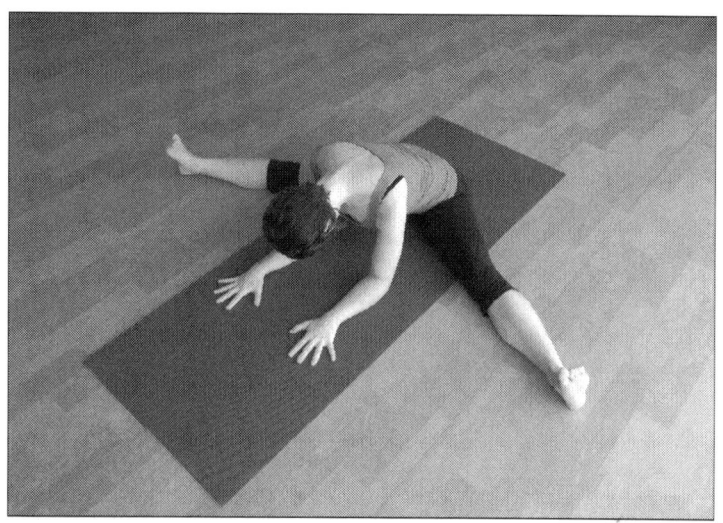

Wide Legged Seated Forward Bend – Upavistha Konasana

Main benefit – Opens the inside of the legs.

1. Start by sitting on the floor or up on some folded blankets (recommend the folded blankets for this one).
2. Bring your legs out wide - to about 90% of your capacity.
3. Start by bringing your hands onto the floor behind your back. Inhale to lengthen your spine and draw your toes back, exhale to use your arms to draw your torso forward and down.
4. If you are new to this stretch then it is probably best to keep your hands behind your back to help you out. If you are more flexible, then bring your hands out in front of your body and use them to help you forward and down.
5. Take your time with this one. Use your breath to support you. You can experiment a little with this one by moving your torso slightly to the left or right to get a different kind of stretch in your inner legs. Stay as long as you like.
6. When ready to come out, simply draw yourself up back into a seated position and slowly draw your legs together.

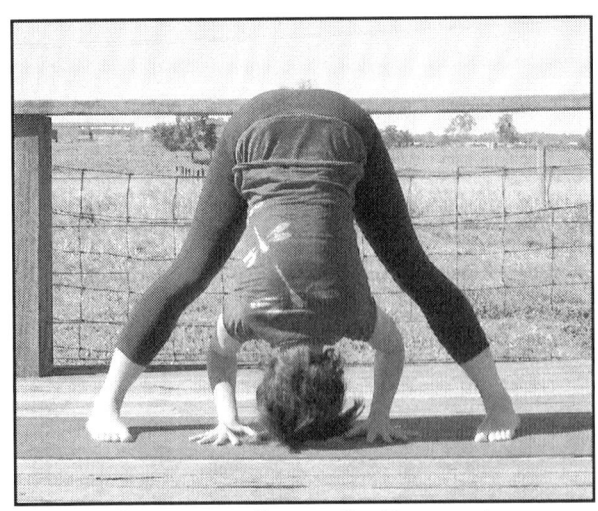

Wide Legged Forward Bend - Prasarita Padottanasana

Main benefit – Opens the inside of the legs and lengthens the back.

1. While standing, step your legs to around 1.5 meters apart (everyone is different so adjust as necessary). Make sure the outsides of your feet are in line with the outsides of the mat or inward just a little – a little pigeon toe is ok.
2. Bring your hands onto your hips, inhale to open your heart to the sky and then exhale to stick your butt out as you draw your chest forward and down toward the floor.
3. Eventually, bring your hands to the mat. If you have trouble reaching the floor with your hands, try widening your legs, and if you still have no luck, bend your knees a little.
4. Bring your hands in between your feet as much as possible, keep your elbows tucked in and then use your arms and hands to draw the top of your head toward the floor.
5. Try keeping your legs activated by pulling up on your kneecaps and trying to stick your buttocks up toward the sky.
6. When you're ready to come out, bend your knees a little, tuck your tail bone under and roll yourself up to a standing position.

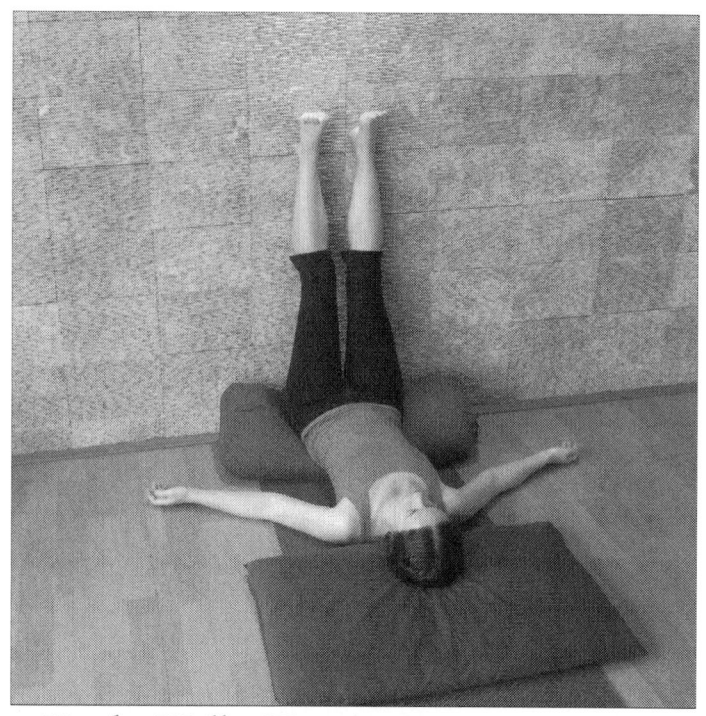

Legs Up the Wall – Viparita Karani
Main benefit – Drains the legs and nourishes the organs.

1. To get into this position can be a bit awkward. To start, the key is to sit up alongside the wall, as close as you can to the wall with one hip.
2. Then, you roll yourself down onto your back and shoot your legs up the wall. Ideally, your buttocks are quite close to the wall, though for people who have tight hamstrings, they will need to come away from the wall so they can get their legs up, their knees will probably be bent, but that's ok. If your hamstrings are ok, wiggle yourself closer to the wall so your buttocks touch the wall.
3. Once you have found a comfortable position, let your arms fall away to the side, close your eyes and just relax with a gentle breath. You can stay here from anywhere between 3-15 minutes.

4. To come out, bend your knees, and then roll to your right side. Wait here for a minute or two so your legs can get some blood back into them before moving or standing. Take your time... if the phone rings or something like that, let it go... Do not rush out of this one.

Variation:
<u>1. If your hamstrings are tight, just wiggle yourself away from the wall until you find a comfortable position</u> where your legs can rest against the wall, your knees will probably be bent, but that's ok.

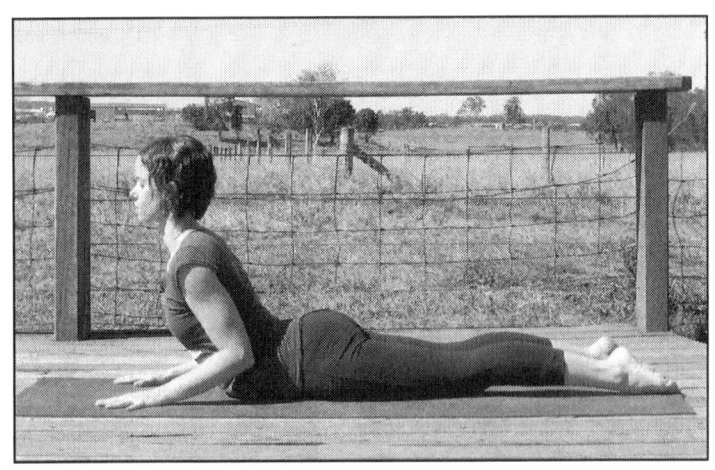

Cobra Pose – Bhujangasana

Main benefit – Provides a gentle back bend which promotes the lower back arch.

1. Start by lying on your belly on the mat.
2. Bring your hands just underneath your shoulders.
3. Raise your chest, head and hands off the floor while looking forward. Get a sense of drawing your shoulder blades together on your back, squeezing your elbows toward each other. This process activates all the back muscles.

Oriental Yoga

4. Place your hands back on the mat and start to raise yourself a little higher into a back bend using your hands. Be careful, listen to your back! Don't worry so much about if your arms are straight or not, it's not important, your back is most important.
5. Only stay up for a breath and then come back down onto your belly.
6. This pose is good to repeat throughout the class.
7. At the beginning of a class or routine only come up a little, when your body is warmed up, then you can go a bit higher.

Other techniques that stimulate the Kidneys and Bladder:

Massage the Feet

1. After a shower is the best time to sit and rub and squeeze your feet with your hands.
2. Start at the inner arches of your feet and use your thumb pads to rub and squeeze.
3. Move onto the belly of the sole of your foot, rubbing and squeezing. I find the thumbs to be the best tools for this. When you find any tender or sore spots, stay on that spot with sustained pressure for a little while before moving on.
4. Make sure you get your toes, rubbing and kind of pinching the tops of your toes.
5. Then, rub the top of your foot and move toward your ankles.
6. Give your ankles a good rub and squeeze before moving to your other foot.

Massage the Ears

This one is great and one of my favorite practices. It is best to do this one daily. It stimulates the brain, the face and the whole body, especially the kidneys.

1. Simply start to rub, squeeze and gently pull your ears. You can be quite strong with your ears, as you want to be able to feel a lot of heat being generated as you do this.

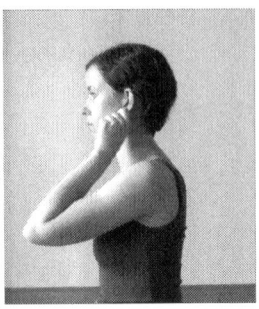

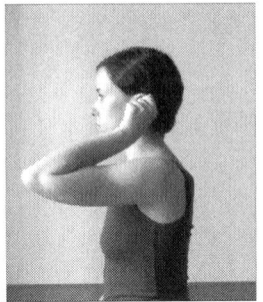

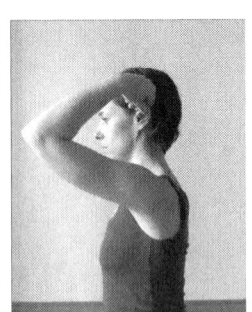

2. Curl open your ears with your fingers and when you find tough bits of cartilage, make sure you get into it and give it a good massage to help break down the stiffness of your ears. Keep breathing, close your eyes if you like, and do this for a good minute or two.
3. Finish by pulling down on your lobs. Relax and have a sip of water. How do you feel?

Hot Water Bottle on the Feet and Lower Back

1. This is especially good if you are prone to lower back pain or getting cold hands and feet easily.
2. Simply place a hot water bottle on your lower back or around your feet as you go to bed or anytime you need some warmth.
3. Practice as often as you like.

Water Element Daily Lifestyle Practices

- Withdraw from excessive activity or overcommitting yourself.

- Early to bed and late to rise (it's the only time of year you can get away with it).

- Spend a little time each day sitting quietly, be still for at least a few minutes each day.

- Enjoy warm, nourishing foods and warm teas. Avoid drinking lots of cold fluids.

- Acknowledge any fears and anxieties that come up and just sit with them, allow them space to exist, don't resist them or run away from them. Look into them deeply…what's there when you get to the depth of them?

- Journal experiences, insights and reflections.

- Cook warming foods and share them with others to help connect to the heart's energy and reduce the feelings of lack of support or isolation.

- Try not to launch any new projects, be patient for now.

- Massage your feet and your loved ones feet often.

- Enjoy hot baths, hot springs.

- **Meditate, Contemplate**

- **Go for walks to move through feelings of stagnation.**

- **It is okay to drink a little red wine with warming herbs.**

Supporting the Other Elements to Assist the Water Element

As outlined in the 5-elements chapter, if we want to balance out the Winter element, we also need to take into consideration the elements that feed and nourish the water element. This is especially the case of illness or any disease related to the kidneys or the bladder. The elements that nourish and support the water element are the Metal element (*Shen* cycle) and the Earth element (*Ko* cycle).

Metal Element Nourishment

- Go for walks to simulate the lungs and circulate energy.
- Let go of any grudges, emotions or memories that tie you to your past.
- Avoid constipation (oats, prunes, linseed, etc).
- Do exercises and movements that lift the arms and stimulate the breath and diaphragm.
- Strip away the non-essentials, refine your character, let go of the past.

Wood Element Stimulation and Harmonization

- Take the time to eat a nourishing breakfast (eg. porridge).
- Eat slowly.
- Engage in activities that help to build a sense of community.
- Do weights and resistance training (morning is best).
- Cultivate trust in the natural flow of life. Avoid doubt or overthinking everything – let it unfold naturally, the universe is

infinitely organized! – Let it do its thing, no need to try and 'work it out' or force it to change.

Food / Oriental Diet Therapy ~ Winter

For *winter,* the following foods and methods are recommended for nourishing and supporting all the organs at this time of year:

Method of Cooking: Soups, stews, baking and slow cooking

Grains: Whole grains, rice, oats

Vegetables: Root vegetables are best – e.g., onions, potatoes, sweet potatoes pumpkin, leeks, etc

Beans and Nuts: Lentils, kidney beans, pine nuts, walnuts and chestnuts

Meat: Lamb, beef, chicken

Herbs and Seasonings: Rosemary, shallots, garlic, onions, chili, cinnamon cloves, black pepper, ginger, fennel, anise, dill and horseradish

Avoid / Reduce
- Salads
- Too many raw foods
- Cold drinks
- Dairy
- Oily, damp foods

- Alcohol (a little warm wine is ok)
- Refined sugars
- White flour

Herbs to Support the Kidneys and Bladder

Here is a list of herbs that support the main organs involved in keeping the kidneys and bladder healthy.

Herbs that nourish and replenish energy in the kidneys and bladder will help keep us steady, calm and courageous. Please seek guidance from a health professional (naturopath, herbalist, Chinese herbalist, Chinese medicine practitioner) for more information about correct dosages or for treating specific conditions.

Ginseng – One of the best for kidney nourishment and tonification. Also supports the spleen and stomach (Earth element) and improves sexual organ function

Astragalus - Tones Qi and supports the immune system

Rehmannia glutinosa – Tones kidneys and helps to reduce hearing loss

Horny Goat Weed (Epimedium sagittatum) – Kidney tonic, aphrodisiac

Dandelion - Detoxes the liver (Wood element), stimulates digestion

Winter Meditations

Taoist Kidney Energy Meditation

Preparation: Sit in a comfortable position. If you are sitting on the floor, I always recommend sitting up on a folded blanket – ideally, you want your knees to be just below your hips. This will help you sit for longer periods without the extra stress to your back. Okay, when you're in a comfortable seated position, place your hands in a comfortable position.

Now close your eyes and settle into a relaxed posture. Find your breath moving through your nostrils and keep watching it. Just keep your attention on your breath, let your thoughts just move through without giving them any attention. Relinquish your mind's thoughts and images as they arise. Come back to your breath with an alert, yet relaxed awareness. Just watch your breath for at least five minutes until your mind starts to settle.

When your mind has settled a little, move your awareness down to your lower back and your lower belly area. As you breathe, feel your breath fill your lower back and simply say something like this to your kidneys, "Thank you, kidneys. Thank you for supporting me, I love and appreciate you and your hard work." The intention is to generate and cultivate appreciation and gratitude toward our kidneys.

You can visualize a deep blue energy being drawn into your lower back and swirling around dissolving any blockages or impurities. Also, set the intention for it to dissolve any fear or anxiety that may be stored there. Be sure to keep a deep exhalation breath going while doing this meditation.

After a few minutes, draw your attention to the point just below your belly button. So as you breathe in, focus your attention on this point and say to yourself, "Hummmmm," and as you breathe out, say to yourself, "Saaaaaaaa."

Do this for a few minutes.

Then begin to visualize a gentle smiling face and then send it down to the area of your lower back and lower belly area. Give thanks to your kidneys by allowing the smiling face to radiate throughout the lower back area.

To complete this mediation, bring your attention back to your breath at your nostrils. Let go of all other practices. Watch your breath until you feel calm and relaxed. Then when ready, open your eyes gently and release your posture.

Wood Element

~ Spring ~

Liver and Gallbladder

Once again, let's have a look at the 5-elements to see where the Wood element sits within this dynamic play.

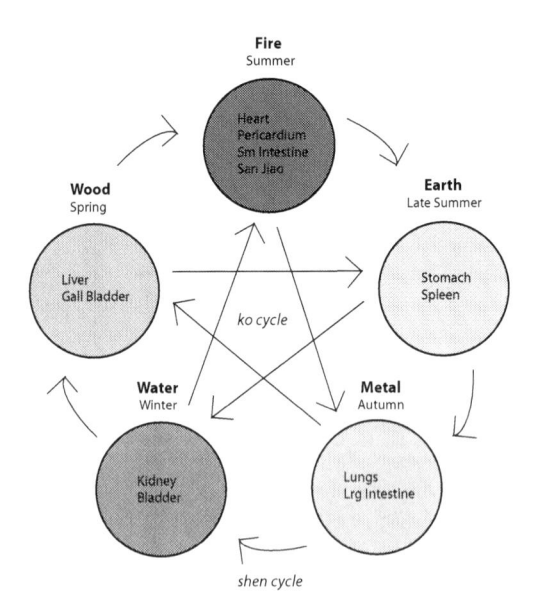

Figure 1.3

When we look at figure 1.3, we can see that the Wood element is supported by the Water element in the *Shen* (nurturing) cycle and the Metal element supports Wood in the *Ko (controlling)* cycle. I will talk a little more about the Water element and Metal element later on.

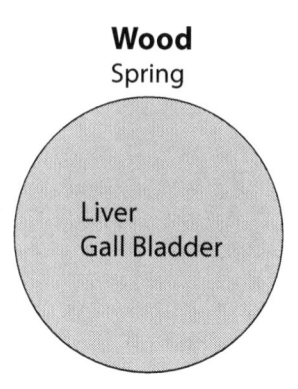

Wood
Spring

Liver
Gall Bladder

Spring is that time of year when new energy, new life and new dreams blossom. As we move out of the colder and more introverted months of winter, we move into the welcome light and warmth of spring. There is freshness and a sense of optimism in the atmosphere as the energy of the sunlight feeds our bodies, our minds and inspires our spirits. The season of spring is associated with the Wood element and is connected to the organs and meridians of the liver and gallbladder. Wood represents new life, rapid growth, flexibility, adaptability and the color green. The liver and the gallbladder are very influential organs as they are largely involved in the process of detoxification, purification, digestion and the energy of expansion and movement. The liver and gallbladder however are easily agitated and this can impact digestion, detoxification, trigger anger and frustration and mild states of depression.

The most common causes of liver and gallbladder energy imbalances are Qi stagnation and an excess of fire in the liver. Qi stagnation is that feeling when you feel stuck in life, of feeling trapped, or that feeling like life just doesn't seem to be flowing very well. It is most often caused by lack of physical body movement such as extended periods of driving cars, sitting at desks or sitting on the couch and generally not moving much. It can also come about when we don't take action on our dreams and visions, opting instead to put up with the daily grind of a boring or unfulfilling job because it appears to be a safe bet.

Excess of liver fire is largely caused by an excess consumption of hot and toxic foods such as alcohol, drugs, smoking, red meat, pharmaceuticals, oily and sugary foods. Any suppressed and oppressed anger also tends to come up a lot during spring. Fortunately, liver and gallbladder imbalances tend to be easy to treat and balance when discovered early. With adjustments in diet, more movement incorporated into one's lifestyle and the letting go of suppressed anger, the liver and gallbladder energy can be effectively cooled and tamed.

Spring is the when yang energy starts expanding and growing and this is why it feels natural to be more upbeat and energized in spring. It's a great time of year to ride the wave of this yang energy by getting up early, engaging in more movement activities like walking or yoga (especially in the mornings) and launching ourselves into new projects.

Spring is the time to feel energized, refreshed, expansive, adaptable, flexible, creative and ready for new opportunities. It's time to launch that business idea you've been planning and thinking about for so long. It's time to start that new exercise class or enroll in that course you've always wanted to take. Spring is one of the best times of year to grow and expand into your higher self.

Wood Organ Physiology

Let's have a look at these organs function from both a western medical perspective and an Oriental medical perspective.

Liver function (Western Medicine)

- The production of bile for the digestion of food and in particular for the digestion of fats
- The production of amino acids (proteins)
- The production of cholesterol and special proteins to assist in the transport of fats around the body.
- The conversion and storing of extra glucose in the form of glycogen that is then converted back into glucose when the body requires more energy.
- The storing and processing of iron for red blood cell production
- The Clearing and cleaning of drugs and toxic substances in the blood
- Removes infectious bacteria from the bloodstream
- Regulates and manages and produces blood clotting factors
- The metabolization of medications into active ingredients

Gallbladder Function (Western Medicine)

- Stores bile (a dark green to yellowish fluid that aids in the digestion of fats that is produced in the liver)
- Secretes bile into the small intestine to aid in digestion and aids in neutralizing acids produced by the stomach

Liver Function (Oriental Medicine)

- Governs the smooth flow of Qi and Blood around the body
- Responsible for filtering, detoxifying, nourishing, replenishing and storing blood
- Governs the tendons and ligaments
- Detoxes the body of toxins
- Related emotion is anger, frustration or their opposite, contentedness

Gallbladder Function (Oriental Medicine)

- Supports the functions of the liver in governing a smooth flow of Qi and blood around the body
- Absorbing and managing excess heat conditions from the liver
- Aids digestion
- Related to indecisiveness and decision making

Physical, Emotional & Spiritual Signs and Symptoms (Oriental medicine)

Liver & Gallbladder <u>In Balance</u>

- Good healthy digestion
- Regular and healthy bowel movements (not too dry, not too wet and one a day before breakfast is ideal)
- Generally in a good and positive mood
- Enjoys moving the body, enjoys exercise, dancing, walking etc.
- Motivated and energized
- Doesn't get angry or frustrated easily
- Is clear and decisive in the decision making process
- Is content and happy with the way life is unfolding
- Willing to launch into new projects
- Is flexible and adaptable to new situations as they arise, (sees them as a healthy challenge rather then an obstacle)
- Healthy eyes with good vision
- Calm and content

Liver & Gallbladder <u>Out Of Balance</u>

- Easy to agitation, frustration & anger
- Feelings of stagnation or being stuck
- Mild depression and moodiness (bipolar related symptoms)
- A poor, sluggish digestion (bloating, excess gas, cramps etc.) or an over stimulated, rapid metabolism (too much fire)
- Can be overweight and slow (not enough heat) or very thin and looks dried out (too much heat)
- Mentally unclear, uncertain and lacks ability to make firm decisions
- Irregular bowel movements eg. Constipation
- Lots of sighs and feelings of, "I can't be bothered" or, "it's too hard!"
- Irregular menstruation
- Tendency to alcohol addiction
- Tendency to drug addiction (marijuana & methamphetamine mainly)
- Lacks energy and motivation
- Ego centric, arrogant
- Stubborn, pig headed and not adaptable to new circumstances
- Intolerant (easily agitated)
- Red face
- Narrow minded – prefers to stick to familiar ways
- Clumsiness
- Shakes or has a tremor in the hands and limbs
- Regular dry, red or irritated eyes, sometimes partnered with vision problems

The Wood Element Meridians

Wood is directly associated with the Liver and Gallbladder organs and meridians. The following pictures and descriptions explore these meridians in further detail.

Liver Meridian

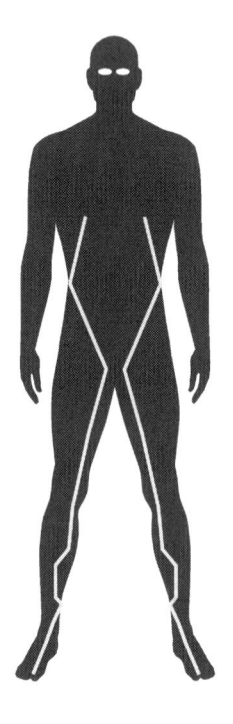

The liver channel begins at the inside of the big toe and travels up the inside of the foot, ankle and leg until it reaches the groin area. It then circulates around the sexual organs and travels up to connect with the liver and gallbladder where it then penetrates deep inside the body. Once it connects up with the liver and gallbladder it travels up to the lungs, mouth and splits into 2 branches to meet the eyes. The two branches then re-join in the forehead area and move inside to the back of the head.

Gallbladder Meridian

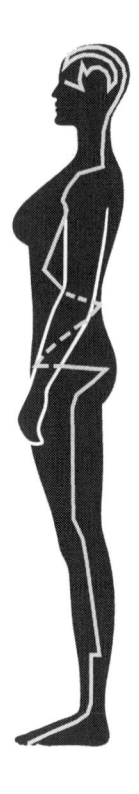

This channel is one of the biggest channels in the body. It begins as two branches that emerge from the outer corners of the eye. An external branch weaves around the face, ear and the side of the head before descending down the side of the body. The other branch crosses the cheek and descends internally to connect with the gallbladder and meet up with the external branch. The branches meet up on the outside of the hip and then the channel travels down the lateral side of the leg, ankle and travels to the tip of the fourth toe. A small branch separates in the fourth toes and travels across to the big toe where it connects with the liver meridian.

Muscles Associated with the Liver

The liver organ and meridian only have two main muscles that are associated with it. Both are involved in the movement and function of the shoulders.

Pectoral Major Sternal

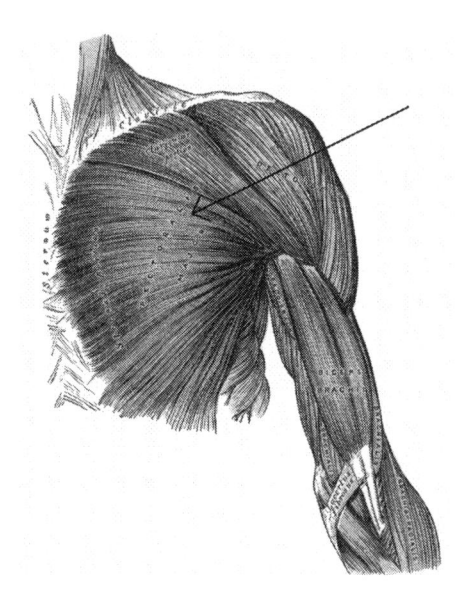

The Pectoral Major Sternal muscle is a large muscle in the upper chest region. The sternal head originates at the sternum and the upper costal (1-6) cartilages of the ribs. The muscle fibers travel across the side of the chest and attach to the lateral lip of intertubercular groove of the humerus.

Rhomboids

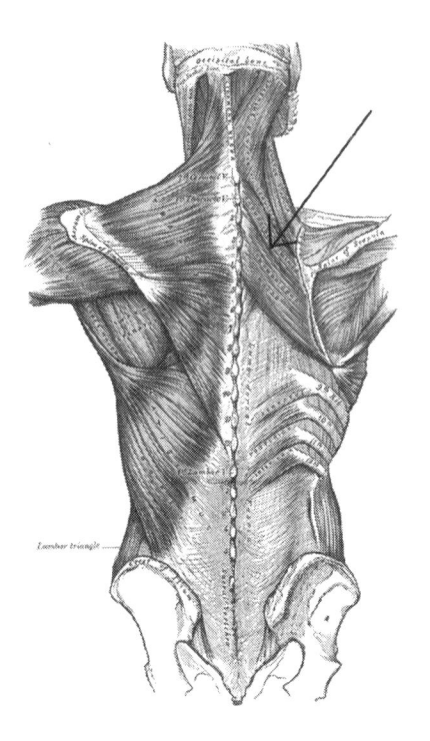

The rhomboids originate on the spinous process of T2 – T5 vertebrae and attach to the medial border of the scapula just inferior to the spine. The rhomboids play a large role in the stabilization of the scapula and therefore play a big role in the overall muscular and skeletal health and balance of the upper back region. The rhomboid muscles can also largely influence tightness in the upper back and spine.

Muscles Associated with the Gallbladder

Anterior Deltoid

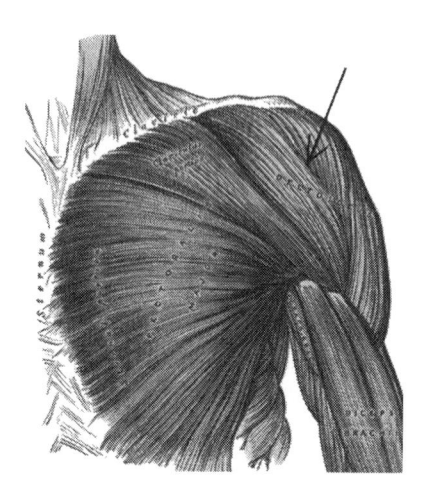

The anterior portion of the deltoid is located on the front of the shoulder. It attaches to the anterior surface of the lateral clavicle and inserts onto the deltoid tuberosity of the humerus.

Popliteus

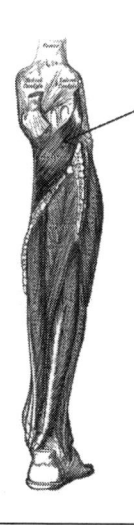

The popliteas muscle is located just below and behind the knee joint. It originates at the lateral surface of the lateral condyle of the femur and attaches to the proximal posterior surface of the tibia.

Asanas (Postures) for Spring

The main aim with the ~~summer~~ asana practices is to open up the gallbladder channel on the side of the body and also stimulate and activate the liver channel on the inside of the legs. Strengthening the upper chest and upper back areas will provide us with more strength while also stimulating digestive fire. Because, the wood element governs the tendons and ligaments, spring is the best time for twisting movements and postures as it helps to keep the ligaments ad tendons healthy. Cooling practices can also be included to help avoid excess fire in the liver.

The following pages provide some asanas that achieve these aims. Incorporate these postures into your asana practice during spring will help to balance the liver and gallbladder.

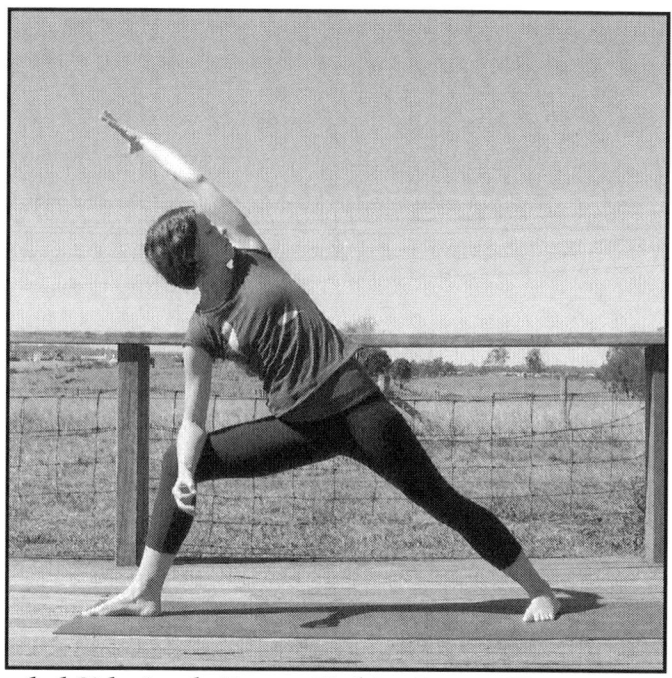

Extended Side Angle Pose – Utthita Parsva Konasana
Main Benefit – Opens the side of body where the gallbladder meridian travels.

1. Extend the legs wide apart and bring your right toe to face down the mat and the back toes to turn out to the side at around 45 degrees.
2. Bring your hands to your hips to start with and start to bend into the front right knee. Make sure your knee is either above your ankle or just behind it, don't let it pass over the ankle as this puts to much stress on the knee joint.
3. Bring your arms up to shoulder height, shoulders relaxed, palms facing down.
4. Now start to reach forward with your right arm, bring your torso forward also, and then place the right elbow onto the knee. Bring the left arms past your ear palm facing down. Look out to the side or up under the arm.

5. Keep your legs strong, draw the belly in, try and relax the upper body.
6. Come out by drawing the arms and torso back to centre, and releasing the legs.
7. Repeat on other side

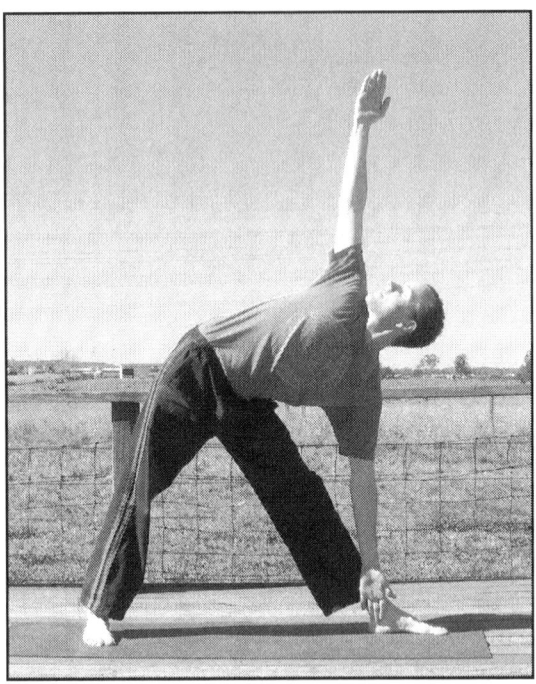

Triangle Pose - Trikonasana
Main Benefit – Opens the side of the body where the gallbladder meridian travels.

1. Bring your feet to about 1 meter apart, not as wide as the warrior 2 pose.
2. Turn the left toes to face the front of the mat and the back toes about 45 to 90 degrees.
3. Bring both arms up to shoulder height, keep your legs straight and then start to bring your arms and torso to the front of the mat as far as you can go.

4. Then simply draw your left arm down onto the left leg, above the ankle a few inches and draw the right arm up to the sky.
5. Keep the chest open. Look to the floor, out to the side or, if the neck is ok try tucking the chin into the right shoulder and look up towards top hand.
6. Keep your legs active by pulling up on the kneecaps. Keep the belly sucked in slightly, steady breathing.
7. Get a sense of pushing the right hip out to the side.
8. Hold for a few breaths and when ready, come out by softening the knees and drawing yourself up.
9. Repeat on the other side.

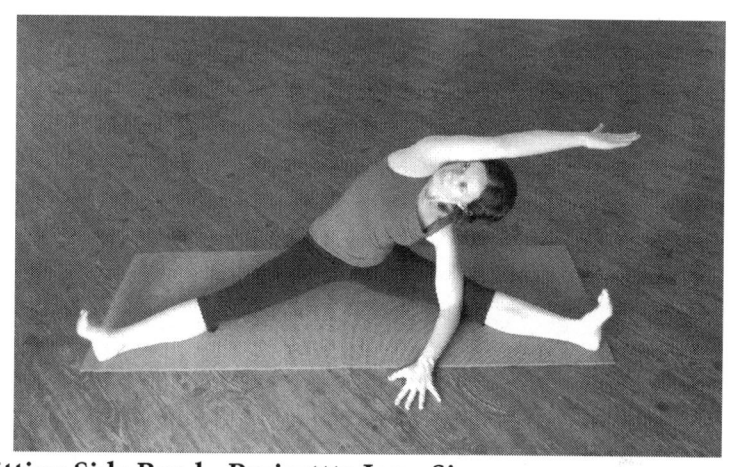

Sitting Side Bend - Parivrttta Janu Sirsasana
Main Benefit – Opens the side of the body where the gallbladder meridian travels as well as opening the liver meridian on the inside of the legs.

1. Bring the left leg straight out to about 45 degrees and the right knee bent with right foot into inner left thigh.
2. Then bring both arms up above the head, draw the belly in and then start to drift the arms and torso over to left leg slightly twisting the torso.

3. Bring the left arm down to the left eg, or floor, wherever it works for you and continue to let the top right arm drift towards the left leg.
4. You can look out to the side or if the neck is ok and you can keep your chest open, try looking up underneath the top arm.
5. Keep your belly slightly drawn in with this pose.
6. Use your exhalation breath to soften into the pose and the inhalation breath to lengthen.
7. Stay for at least a few good, deep breaths, close your eyes if you like.
8. To come out simply draw your torso back towards centre and rest the arms.
9. Repeat to the other side.

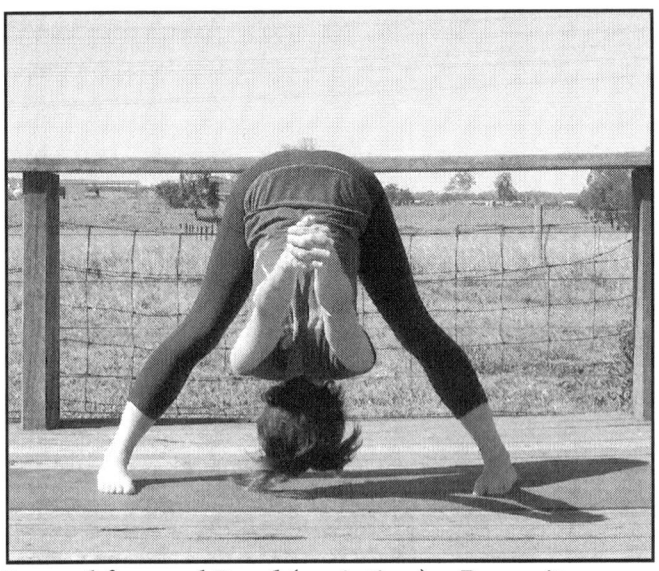

Wide Legged forward Bend (variation) – Prasarita Padottanasana

Main Benefit – A cooling pose that opens the channels on the inside of the legs, arms and shoulders.

1. Take a wide legged stance with toes both facing to the side of the room.

Oriental Yoga

2. Interlace your hands behind your back while upright. Then inhale, lengthen your spine upwards and then as you exhale start to stick your buttocks out behind and draw the torso forward and down while letting the arms drift up behind you.
3. Allow a few breaths to settle into this pose – keep breathing and relax your head.
4. When you're ready to come up, bend your knees slightly, and imagine someone is behind you pulling you up by your arms bringing you upright.
5. Relax the arms and release the legs.

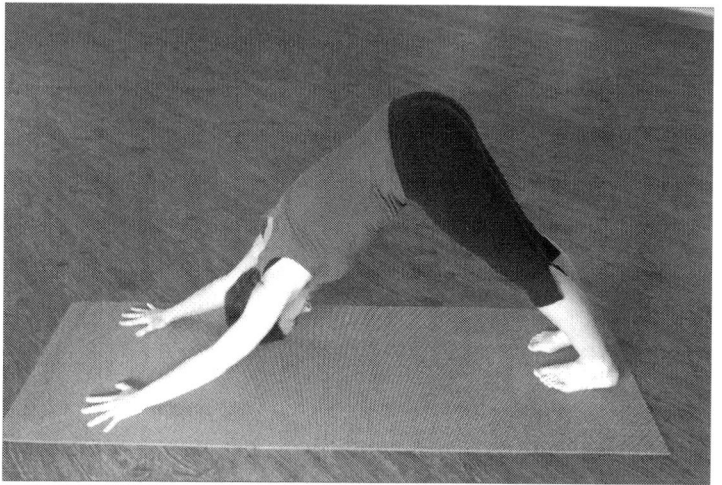

Down Facing Dog – Adho Mukha Svanasana
Main benefit – Strengthens and opens the arms, chest, shoulders and the back of the legs.

1. Come onto all fours with hands underneath the shoulders and knees under the hips. Spread your fingers wide.
2. Tuck the toes under, start to extend the arms and start bringing the knees off the floor.
3. Come to extend the arms, and start to work the kegs straight. Try to bring the weight back into your legs and not so much into your arms.
4. Look to the floor just under your belly button.

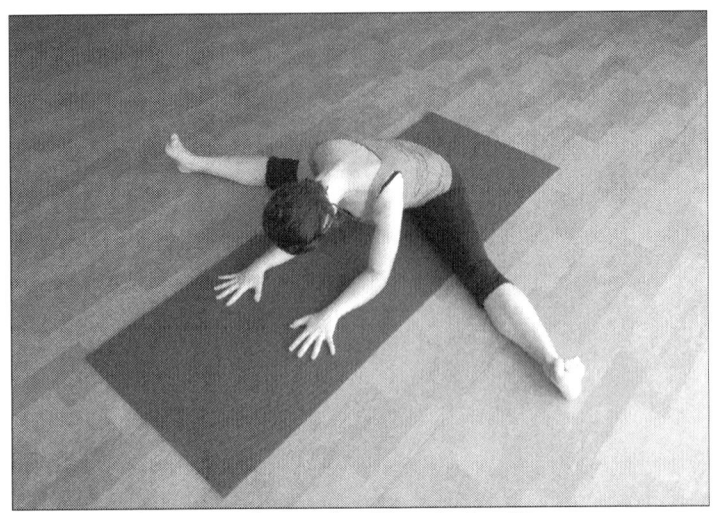

Wide Legged Forward Bend – Upavistha Konasana

Main benefit – Opens the channels on the inside of the legs and helps to re-orientate the hips.

1. Come to sit on your mat and spread the legs wide to about 90% of your capacity. If you have difficulty with this posture and find your back rounding and buttocks tucking under then place one or two folded blankets under your buttocks (slightly raising the hips in seated postures dramatically helps those with tight hips and hamstrings)
2. Now, bring your hands behind you onto the floor to help support a straight back. Sit up as straight as you can to get length in your spine and upper body.
3. Draw the toes back towards the head and gently pull the kneecaps up to activate your leg muscles.
4. When you are ready use your hands that are behind you to draw your chest forward. You can stay here if you feel a strong stretch already.
3. If you want to go further bring the hands in front of you and while keeping the lower back long, allow your chest to lower towards the floor.

4. Make sure you keep your breath flowing and stay at the sot where you feel a good stretch occurring. Stay for at least 2 minutes, making slight adjustments as you deepen into the pose.
5. When you are ready to come out, use your hands to slowly draw your torso back up to a seated position. Release your legs by drawing them together and wrapping your arms around the legs to give yourself a hug.

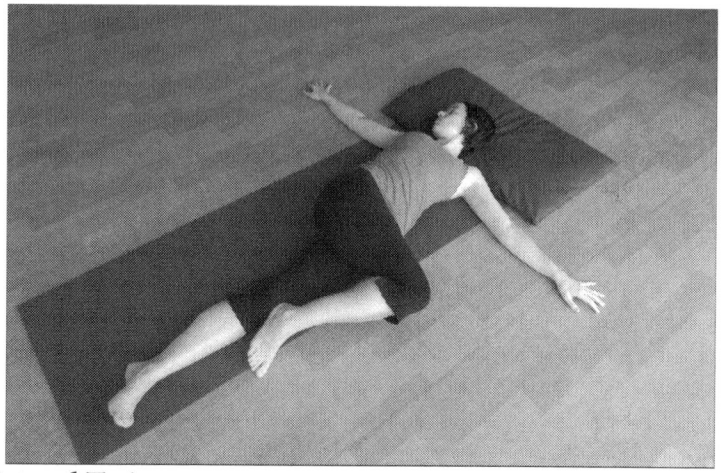

Natural Twist
Main Benefit – Squeezes the organs to support detoxification as well as stretching the ligaments and tendons.

This pose usually requires no support or props, though some people benefit from having something under the bent leg. Try it without the support first, but if it feels too strenuous or your breath is halted, then you may need to use a bolster or pillow under the bent leg. Have a bolster or pillow nearby just in case.

1. To get into this position, first just lay flat out onto the floor.
2. Bring the left arm out to the side at about shoulder height, keeping your elbow bent or your arm straight; whichever feels better and whatever you have the space for.

3. Bend your left knee so that the knee joint is sitting comfortably at about ninety degrees.
4. Bring your right hand to your left knee and start to guide the knee across your body so that you come into a twist.
5. Let the leg come as far over towards the floor as possible. It you start straining, then wither back off a bit, or bring a bolster or pillow under that bent leg so it can come to relax.
6. Find a comfortable position in which you can breathe smoothly.
7. If your neck is okay, try looking back over your left arm.
8. Stay for at least one minute.
9. Release by bringing the bent leg back up to the middle and straightening out both legs. Rest for a moment, then go to the other side.
10. Repeat steps 2 – 8 with the opposite arms and legs.

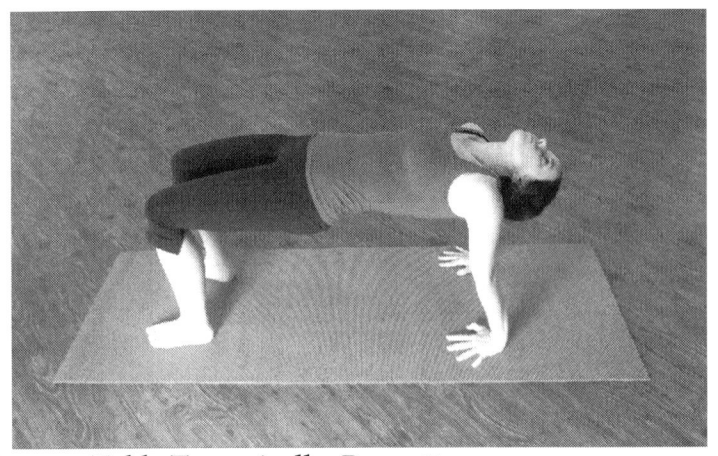

Reverse Table Top – Ardha Purvottanasana
Main Benefit – Strengthens the back of the body and opens the channels on the arms and on the front of the body.

1. Come to sit on your mat, with your knees bent and feet flat on the mat.
2. Bring your hands just behind you, fingers pointing forwards.

Oriental Yoga

3. Start by raising the buttocks just off the floor.
4. If ok, raise the hips all the way so they are in line with your knees and shoulders.
5. Let your head rest back into the fold of the neck.
6. Get a sense of the shoulder working down away from the head. Allow the elbows to have a tiny bend in them, avoid hyperextending the elbow joint.
7. Plant your fingers and toes into the floor.
8. Connect with your breath and hold for around 5 long steady breaths.
9. To come out slowly lower your buttocks first, the head will naturally roll up without any effort.
10. Come to sit back on the mat.

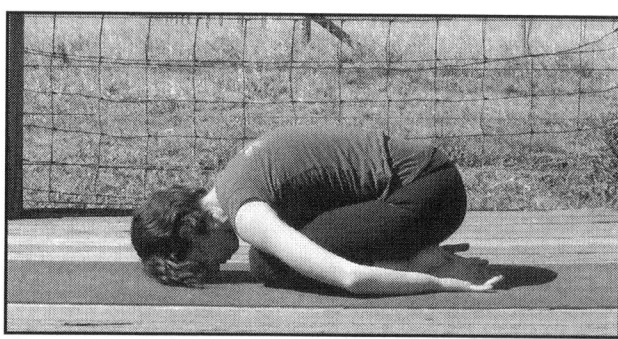

Child's Pose – Balasana

Main benefit – A cooling pose to calm the mind, draws energy inwards and softens the back.

1. Sit on your heels, feet flat in the seiza position (traditional Japanese posture of sitting on the heels). If it's too much on your ankles or knees, try placing a blanket under your feet and knees. If this doesn't work for you, then just come down into a cross-legged seated position.
2. From here, simply draw your torso down toward the floor. Rest your forehead on the floor. Relaxed arms can be out in front or down the side.

3. Close your eyes and take a few breaths, relax your back and shoulders.
4. When you're ready to come out, simply draw your torso back up to sit on your heels or on the floor.
- The child's pose can be done anytime you feel like you need to have a rest or break, especially in yoga class.

Other techniques that regulate the Liver and Gallbladder:

Pummeling the Body

This is a common practice in the arts of Qi gong and tai chi. It involves simply the act of drumming and pummeling various parts of the body with loose fists. If you have ever travelled to Korea, Japan or China you will often see older people in the park practicing this pummeling technique. The primary benefit and purpose of this practice is to free up any energy stagnation in the system. Often after a pummeling the body for 5 – 10 minutes the body will feel very "buzzy" and it also produces a very calming affect. It is often a useful and effective technique to reduce pain related symptoms because in Oriental medicine pain is primarily seen as the stagnation of Qi energy. Therefore freeing up any Qi energy stagnation will relieve pain related symptoms.

Here is some instruction on how to pummel your arms and your legs to remover energy stagnation:

Shoulders and Arms

1. Hold a loose fist with your right hand and gently, yet firmly (we want the body to shake to the pressure of the pummel but we don't want to produce pain) and start to pummel into the muscle between the tip of your left shoulder and your neck (the trapezius muscle).

Oriental Yoga

2. After a minute start to pummel down the outside of your left arm. When you reach the hand turn the hand over and gently pummel up the inside of the left arm.
3. Go up and down the arm about 2 or 3 times and then swap hands and do the same thing on to the right shoulder and arm.

Legs

1. Bring both hands into a loose fist and start to pummel the top of the buttocks. Allow your arms to be as relaxed as you can, keep the elbows soft as you pummel.
2. After a minute or two start to slowly move your pummeling down the outside of your legs. Down the thighs, avoid the knees and pummel down the outside of the calves.
3. When you reach the feet bring the hands to the inside of the ankles, a little softer now as you begin to pummel up the insides of the legs. The inside of the legs is generally more sensitive then the outside of the legs so take it easier when working with the inside of the legs.
4. Pummel slowly all the way up to the inner thighs and then move the hands back around to the top of the buttocks to do another round.
5. Complete 2-3 rounds and then stand, release your hands, close your eyes and just take a moment for your body to settle. Can you feel it buzzing?

Massage the Organs

Massaging the organs stimulates and triggers the organs into action. It also helps to squeeze toxins out of the system.

1. There is an easy way to massage the organs by lying on a yoga mat on your belly. Relax your head either to the side or bring both hands up to under your chin and place your head on your hands.

2. Bend your knees and let your feet dangle in the sky.
3. Then gently start to make circles in the air with your feet. (feet going in the same direction). You should feel a pressure in the belly area and it will move around your belly area as you move your feet. Continue for about a minute and then rest

There are plenty of other ways to massage the organs but it is advised to either attend a suitable yoga class, a workshop or get guidance from a health professional as to how to go about it.

Qi Gong & Free Flowing Movements

The movements of Qi Gong are perfect for liver energy. The liver loves movement and it especially loves smooth movements, which are found in Qi Gong. Qi Gong movements take some time to get used to and therefore it is advisable to attend some classes to get the feel of it. Once you get the feel of it, you can return to it at any point and explore it in your own way. If you are a yoga or movement teacher, incorporating some forms of Qi Gong movements during spring will add more power to your classes and it will help smooth out everybody's liver and gallbladder energy.

Qi stagnation is one of the common causes that lead people to mild depressive symptoms. It can easily and effectively be relieved through removing stagnation through Qi Gong and most martial arts practices. Also, going out for regular walks every day will dramatically improve their overall wellbeing.

Wood Element Daily Lifestyle Practices

- Early to rise and go for a walk or practice some yoga / Qi Gong / exercise to get the Qi and blood moving

- Lemon water on waking to flush the liver

- In bed before 11pm

- Take up a new movement class or incorporate more movement into your day.

- Write up and brainstorm things you want to work on and bring into your life and throw out the things that don't support that vision.

- Spring clean. Clean out your bedroom, house, car etc. Throw away the non-essentials. Be ruthless!

- Spend more time in nature and being in green environments.

- Be creative at night. Don't watch the news or get work serious in the evening, instead dance, move, go to a yoga class, make music.

- Be open to new people and opportunities as they arise. Allow yourself to be open and flexible and adaptable.

- Avoid or reduce those things that generate excess heat in the liver e.g. alcohol, drugs, BBQ'd foods, smoking, pharmaceuticals. This will help reduce the intensity and frequency of anger outbursts.

- Meditation, acupuncture, massage (helps Qi to become smooth & cools the liver)

- Ride the wave of new energy and use it to learn new things or launch into new projects.

Supporting the Other Elements to Assist the Wood Element

As outlined in the 5 elements chapter, if we want to balance out the Wood element, we also need to take into consideration the elements that feed the Wood element which are Water (*Shen* cycle) and Metal (*Ko* cycle). This is especially the case of any illness or any disease related to the liver or gall bladder.

Water Element Stimulation and Harmonization

- Keep cool. Cold showers and laying down to rest in the hottest part of the day can help to keep you cool
- Meditation, gentle yoga stretching, stillness and quiet time
- Good quality sleep
- Look after your kidneys with good quality water and keep hydrated
- Eat root vegetables

Metal Element Nourishment

- Wake early to get fresh energy into the lungs
- Go for walks to simulate the lungs and circulate energy
- Let go of any grudges, emotions or memories that tie you to your past
- Avoid constipation (oats, prunes, linseed, etc)
- Do exercises and movements that lift the arms and stimulate the breath and diaphragm
- Strip away the non-essentials, refine your character, let go of the past

Food / Oriental Diet Therapy ~ Spring

For *spring*, the following foods and methods are recommended for nourishing and supporting all of the organs at this time of year:

Method of Cooking: Lightly cooked foods (steaming, poaching, stir-frying), small amounts of raw foods. Soups, stews, congees and casseroles are advised for those with any digestive problems or are ill or weak in any way.

Grains: rice, barley, oats, spelt, quinoa, wheat bran

Vegetables: onions, asparagus, cabbage, cauliflower, broccoli, brussels sprouts, beetroot, carrots, celery, turnip, pumpkin, leafy vegetables, sweet potato

Fruits: grapefruit, tangerines, peach, strawberries, figs

Nuts, Seeds and Beans: sunflower seeds, sesame seeds, adzuki beans, black beans, string bean, tofu, soybean and only a little amount of pine nuts and almonds

Meat: fish (mackerel, tuna, halibut), chicken, turkey, a little beef or lamb preferably well cooked in a soup or congee

Herbs and Seasonings (only if lacking fire or feeling stagnant): black pepper, ginger, garlic, cinnamon, nutmeg, and fennel

In Case of Energy (Qi) Stagnation: Small quantities of wine and/or coffee (black and one a day) can be helpful to stimulate digestion, move Qi, blood and support healthy bowel movements.

Avoid / Reduce
- Cheese, cream, ice-cream
- Pizzas
- Deep Fried Foods
- Excessively spicy foods
- Refined sugars, artificial preservative and artificial colorings
- Beer
- Margarines
- Excessive amounts of red meat and BBQ'd foods

Herbs to Support the Liver and Gallbladder

Here is a list of herbs that support the main organs involved in keeping the liver and gallbladder healthy. Taking herbs and supplements alongside a healthy lifestyle that incorporates yoga will provide more effective results.

Please seek guidance from a health professional (naturopath, herbalist, Chinese herbalist, Chinese medicine practitioner) for more information about correct dosages or for treating specific conditions.

Mary's Thistle – The kingpin of liver tonics, this herb helps cleanse the liver of toxins, helps to regenerate damaged liver tissue and supports digestion

Dandelion Root – Helps cleanse the liver and stimulates the flow of bile

Chicory Root – Helps cleanse the liver

Peppermint – A cooling digestive stimulant and helps support the liver in the breakdown of fats

Fish Oils and other sources of Omega 3's – Helps to lubricate the tendons and ligaments around the joints

Gingko Biloba – Supports the efficient transport of qi and blood around the body

Spring Meditations

<u>Letting Go Meditation</u>

Preparation: Sit in a comfortable position. If you are sitting on the floor, I always recommend sitting up on a folded blanket – ideally, you want your knees to be just below your hips. This will help you sit for longer periods without the extra stress in your back.

When you are in a comfortable seated position, place your hands in a comfortable position. I generally recommend interlacing your fingers and placing them on your lap or just in front of your lap, or simply place one palm on top of the other. Ok, now close your eyes and settle into a relaxed posture. Find your breath moving through your nostrils and gentle keep your attention on it. Let your thoughts just move through your mind without giving them any attention. Relinquish your mind's thoughts and images as they arise. If you get distracted, no matter; gently come back to your breath with an alert, yet relaxed awareness.

1. Now, when you feel settled, have a little think about something that happened to you today, or yesterday, that annoyed or frustrated you. Bring it up in your mind.
2. Now notice how it feels in your body. Where do you feel it the most?
3. Stay with it for a moment and be aware of these sensations like you are watching them from a distance.
4. Now, but instead of resisting it, as we normally tend to do, this time allow it to "run its course" without any resistance in you. Relax into it, no matter how pleasant or unpleasant.

5. Keep watching the sensations, the feelings the emotions swim around inside but do not engage in them, just watch them and relax into it.
6. Eventually, in a matter of minutes usually the intensity of it fades away into insignificance. How long does it last before it starts to fade away?
7. Continue to be free of resistance until most of the feelings have subsided.
8. When you are ready to come out of it, open your eyes and relax your posture.

If you feel up to the challenge you can always bring to mind another past event that brings up in you feelings of anger or frustration. And again repeat the process. Watching the sensations in the body, and then letting them run their course without any resistance until they eventually run out of stream.

After some time of practicing this technique you can apply it to gradually larger and larger events or circumstances where it brings up intense emotions, feelings and sensations in your body. This is a very powerful technique that can help us all to relieve any oppressed and suppressed emotions, in particular anger, fear and grief.

Walking Meditation

Walking mediation is suitable for wood element in particular because the liver energy loves to move. We can use slow and mindful walking as a way to train our minds and enhance our ability to be in the present moment.

There are four primary movements of the feet when we walk and these are the movements that we focus on when we practice walking mediation.

1. In standing, allow your arms to rest by your sides. Generally the gaze is diagonally downwards to the ground about 10 meters in front. This helps to reduce mental activity and it also reduces distractions in the field of vision.
2. Bend your knees slightly. Relaxed posture.
3. On the 1st movement of the foot - Start to slowly raise the right foot off the floor
4. On the 2nd movement – slowly glide the right foot forward through the air
5. On the 3rd movement – slowly place the right heel of the foot on the floor and start to shift your body weight forward onto the right foot
6. On the 4th movement – come to place the ball of the foot onto the ground and draw all your body weight forward onto the right foot
7. Now, we move to the left foot and go through the 1-4 movements again on this foot.
8. The challenge of this meditation is to remain completely aware of every one of the 4 movements without getting distracted or rushing through it.

Try practicing this for at least 5 minutes and work your way up to 10 minutes per session. This meditation is a great complement to other meditational practices because it develops focus, concentration and mindfulness.

Fire Element

~ Summer ~

Heart and Small Intestine

The last element we need to look at is the Fire element. Let's have a look at the 5-elements to see where the Fire element sits within this dynamic play.

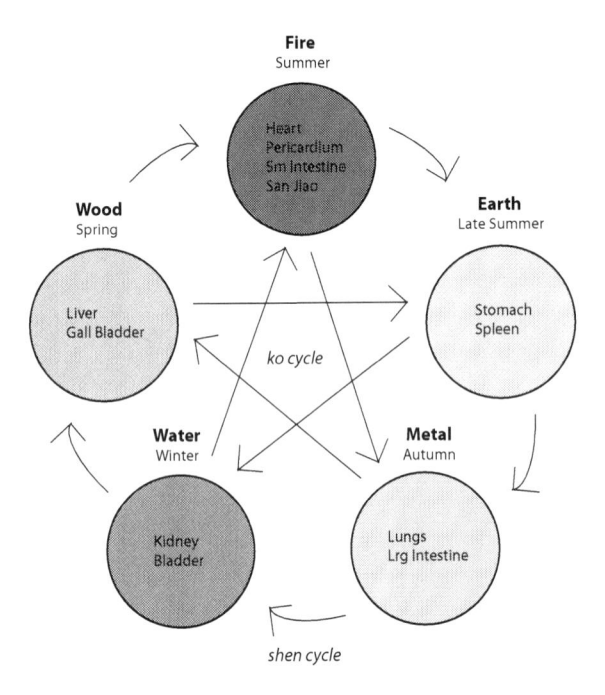

Figure 1.3

When we look at figure 1.3, we can see that the Fire element is supported by the Wood element in the *Shen* (nurturing) cycle and the Water element supports Fire in the *Ko (controlling)* cycle. I will talk a little more about the Wood element and Water element later on in this chapter.

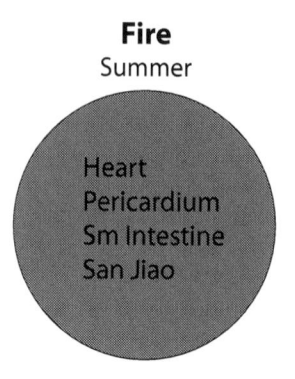

Fire
Summer

Heart
Pericardium
Sm Intestine
San Jiao

Summer (Fire element) is the hottest and driest time of year. It's that time when the days are long and hot and the nights are short and warm. In the traditional system, the Fire element is the only element that consists of four organs and one of those organs is technically not even an organ (San Jiao). In order to simplify, we will focus on the two primary organs in the Fire element which is the heart and small intestine. The heart has great significance in Oriental medicine as it is often described as the home and sanctuary of the mind and the spirit.

Summer is the perfect expression of yang energy and because of the nature of yin and yang, when any extreme is experienced, as exemplified by the intense summer yang days, the tendency is to seek out yin activates such as eating cooler foods and seeking shelter from the sun as a way to restore some kind of balance.

Also in summer there is a tendency reduce the intake of food because there is already an excess amount of energy and heat in the environment, therefore the body doesn't require as much energy from food.

The emotions associated with the Fire element are love, joy, excitement and hate. When inspiration flows, love and joy also flow. However, when there is a disturbance in the heart energy, hatred and intolerance replace the flow of inspiration.

Summer is the time to feel <u>inspired, joyful, loving, compassionate and open to life in all its expressions.</u> It's time to dream big, to have fun, to motivate and connect with others and support their dreams and visions. Summer is an exciting time and a great time of year to get out more and party, to stay up late dancing during the warm nights.

Fire Organ Physiology

Let's have a look at these organs function from both a western medical perspective and an Oriental medical perspective.

Heart function (Western Medicine)

- Pumps blood throughout the entire body
- Has 4 main parts or chambers: right atrium, left atrium, right ventricle, left ventricle
- The right atrium receives blood from the veins and pumps it to the right ventricle
- The left atrium receives oxygenated blood from the lungs and pumps it to the left ventricle
- The right ventricle receives blood from the right atrium and pumps it to the lungs to be oxygenated
- The left ventricle is the strongest chamber and pumps the oxygen rich blood throughout the body

Small Intestine Function (Western Medicine)

- Absorbs most of the nutrients from what we eat and drink

Heart Function (Oriental Medicine)

- Pumps blood throughout the entire body
- Controls Blood and Vessels
- Houses the *Shen* (spirit and mind)
- Heart supports speech and appropriateness
- Contributes to the regulation of overall body temperature

Small Intestine Function (Oriental Medicine)

- Absorbs most of the nutrients from what we eat and drink
- Separates the pure aspects of the food and drink from the impure

Physical, Emotional & Spiritual Signs and Symptoms (Oriental medicine)

Heart & Small Intestine <u>In Balance</u>

- Good healthy digestion
- Generally in a good and positive mood
- Appropriate and considerate
- Easy to sleep and easy rest
- Easy to inspire and easy to inspire others
- Motivated and energized
- Able to have fun and laugh
- Enjoys connecting with others
- A sense of inner joy and peacefulness
- Doesn't depend on external circumstances for happiness.
- Able to love thy self and love others without judgment
- Warm hearted, compassionate

Heart and Small Intestine <u>Out Of Balance</u>

One extreme is that the fire is deficient and lacking. The tendency of this imbalance is that one feels heavy, slow, depressive and unmotivated. The other extreme is one who has too much fire and heat. The tendency of this imbalance is that the person is very thin, fast, neurotic and mentally unstable.

- Anxiety, depression, moody
- Insomnia (inability to fall to sleep easily and/or wakes often after a few hours)

- Lacks the ability to feel love openly and honestly
- Heart palpitations
- Always feelings of uneasiness, instability
- Inappropriate social behavior
- Excessive nervous laughter
- Poor sluggish digestion or digestion is too fast
- Emotionally sensitive or not sensitive enough – can take things too personally and over react or can be emotionally cold, lack compassion and be 'heartless'.
- Can be very serious, finds it difficult to relax and have fun
- Stressed out, workaholic, easy to drug addictions, gambling etc.
- Experiences hate for oneself and hate for the world
- Sexual deviancy / sexual misconduct e.g. pedophilia

The main causes of imbalance:
The heart (*Shen*) is sensitive and can be easily disturbed by having too many late nights without sleep, excessive stress, the continuous oppression and suppression of feelings, ongoing intoxicant abuse, severe traumatic events and from the overstimulation of the eyes e.g. playing computer games for long periods. Basically, anything that triggers the heart rate to beat fast for extended periods of time will disturb psychological health and balance.

The Fire Element Meridians

Fire is associated with the Heart and Small Intestine organs and meridians, so let's have a look at where these meridians travel throughout the body.

Heart Meridian

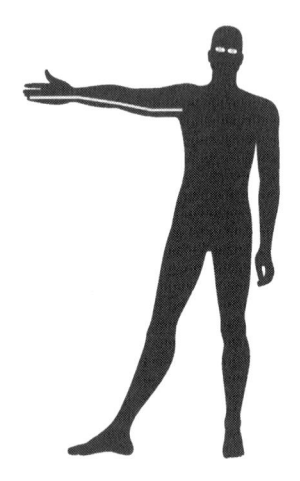

The heart channel originates in the heart organ itself. One branch moves downwards through the diaphragm to the small intestine. Another branch moves upwards through the throat connects at the tongue and travels up to the eyes. The third branch moves through the lungs before it comes to the surface just under the armpit. From the armpit it moves down the inside of the arms passing the inner end of the elbow crease. It continues down the inside of the arm, across the palm and finishes at the inside tip of the little finger.

Small Intestine Meridian

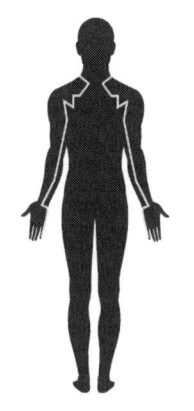

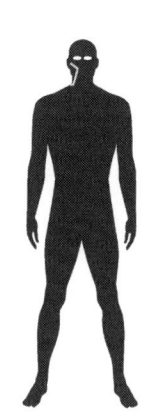

This channel begins on the outside corner of the little fingernail. It travels up the outer edge of the hand to the wrist where it starts to travel up the forearm. It passes the elbow at the "funny bone" as it continues up the back of the arm and heads to the back of the shoulder joint. It then moves in a somewhat jiggered fashion across the shoulder blades, before travelling over the top of the shoulders to the hollow above the collarbone on the front of the body. An internal branch heads inwards to the heart and down the esophagus to the stomach and small intestine. The superficial branch travels from the collarbone up the side of the neck and over the cheeks and draws back towards the ears where it finishes.

Muscles Associated with the Heart

The heart organ and meridian only has one main muscle that is associated with it.

Subscauplaris

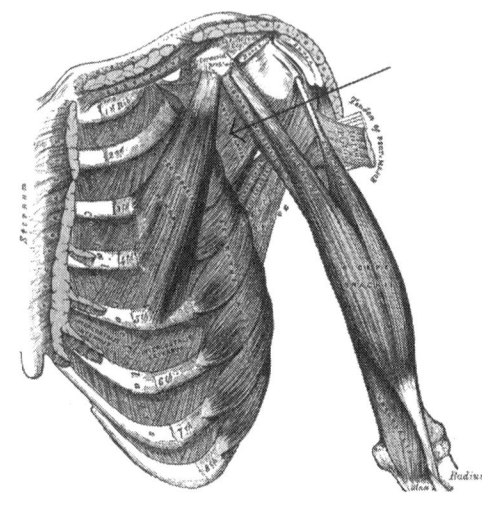

The subscapular muscle is a large triangular muscle that lies underneath the scapula bone (shoulder blade) on the back of the body. It originates from the medial and lower groove on the axillary border of the scapula. It inserts as a tendon onto the lesser tubercle of the humerus and the anterior part of the shoulder joint capsule.

Muscles Associated with the Small Intestine

Most of the muscles associated with the spleen are in the back and indicate that healthy and active back muscles not only support a healthy spine but also support a health digestive system.

Transverse Abdominus

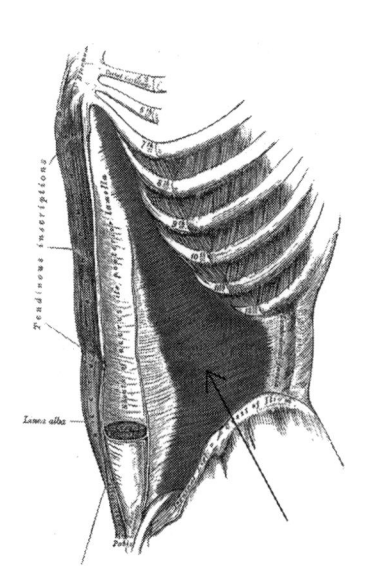

The Transverse Abdominus is one of the main muscles involved in the core. It originates from a variety of locations including the iliac crest, the inguinal ligament, thoracolumbar fascia and the costal cartilages of ribs 7-12. The fibers travel crossways and diagonally to attach to the xiphoid process, the linea albla, the public crest and the pectin pubis.

Rectus Abdominus

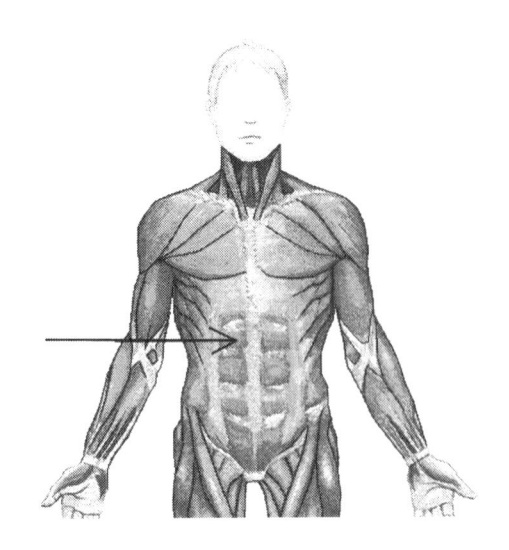

Another group of muscles involved in the core the rectus abdominals originates at the crest of the pubis and attaches to the costal cartilage of ribs 5-7 and the xiphoid process of the sternum. It consist of the paired muscles running vertically, speared by a midline band of connective tissue called the linea alba giving it a ridged or "6-pack" look.

Quadriceps

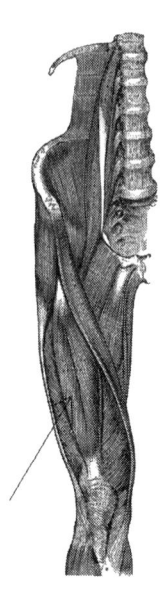

The quadriceps is a large and powerful muscle group that involves 4 main muscles at the front of the thigh. It originates on the lower border of the iliac spine and from the surface of the femur bone. It inserts onto the tibial tuberosity, the patellar tendon and the patella.

Asanas (Postures) for Summer

The main aim with the summer asana practices is to open the heart and small intestine channels on the front of the body and on the arms, while strengthening and toning the muscles involved in the core. Cultivating power and strength in the legs also helps to ground the system's energy into the earth and builds fire for digestion. Cooling practices can also be included to avoid excess fire in the system and to help calm the spirit/mind. Below are some asanas that achieve this aim.

Incorporate these postures into your asana practice during summer to stimulate the inner fire and help balance the mind.

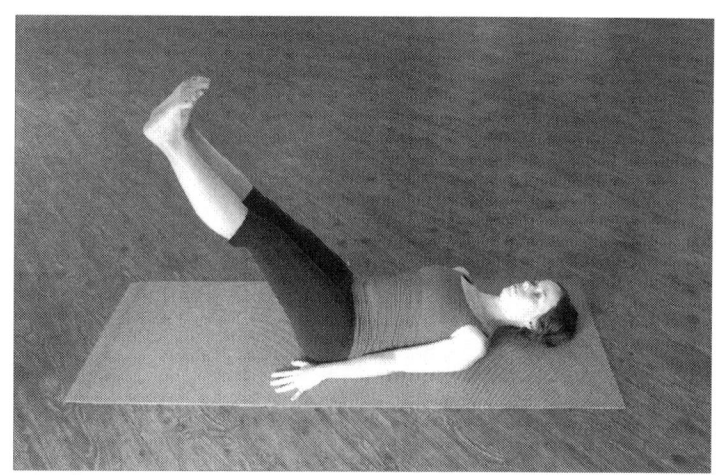

Leg Lifts
Main benefit – Activates and strengthens the abdominal core muscles.

1. Lie on your back on the mat, arms down the side of the body, palms down.
2. Bend your knees to help you draw your feet up into the sky directly above your hips.
3. Pull back on your toes, activate your thigh muscles by pulling up on the kneecaps.
4. Start slowly by lowering your legs towards the floor. Keep them straight and activated the whole time!
5. As soon as your lower back start to come off the mat that's the indicator to stop and slowly return your legs up to the vertical position.
6. Repeat the process of slowly lowering the legs and raising them steadily back up about 8-10 times. If you get really tired, then rest the legs for a moment but make sure you do the full 8-10 repetitions.

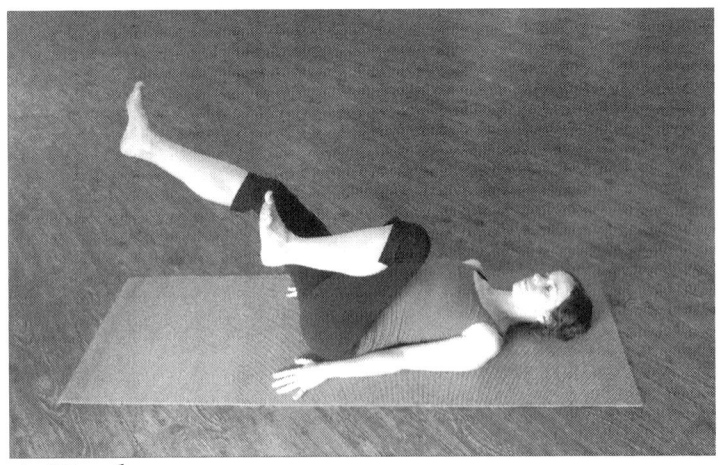

Yogic Bicycle
Main benefit – Activates and strengthens the abdominal core muscles

1. Lie on your back on the mat, arms down the side of the body, palms down.
2. Bend your knees and begin by placing your feet into a position similar to that of riding a bicycle.

3. Pull back on the toes to keep your legs active and start to make rotations in the sky like you are riding a bicycle.
4. Keep it going for at least 1-2 mintues. You want to generate that feeling of fire and heat in the belly region.
5. Keep going,. Eventually start to slow down the cycle movement and then move your legs in the opposite direction as if you are riding a bicycle in reverse.
6. When you are ready to stop, slow down the movements and then bend your knees into your chest to release.

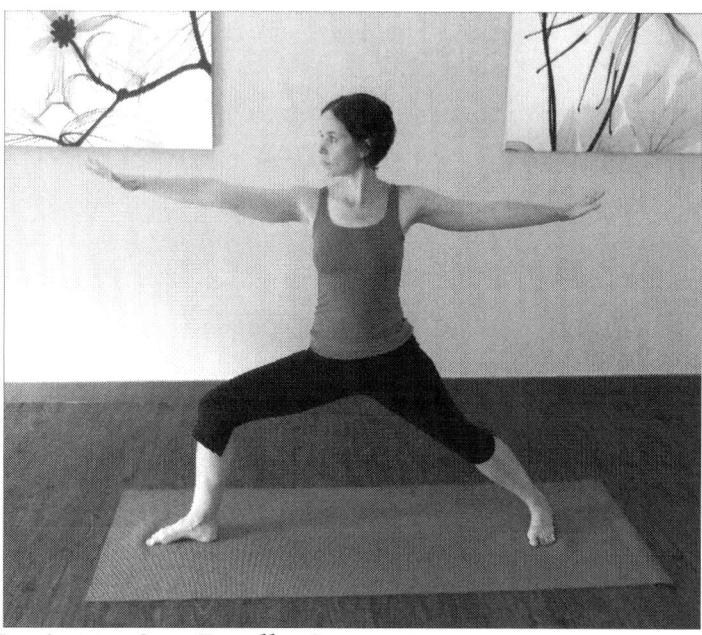

Warrior 2 – Setu Bandha Sarvangasana
Main benefit – Strengthens the legs and opens the arm channels.

1. Bring your legs wide apart. Turn your left toes to the front of the mat and your back toes around 45 degrees.
2. Bring your hands onto your hips to start with and sink into your left knee, making sure that the left knee remains either above or just behind the ankle joint.
3. Get solid in the legs, tuck the belly in slightly

4. Then extend the arms out at shoulder height with the palms down. Soften the shoulders and the elbows so that the Qi can move easily.
5. Gazing down the front arm –extending your Qi through your eyes.
6. Spread the fingers wide to encourage the Qi to move into the hands.
7. You can pull the finger back towards the body to emphasis the Qi in the wrists and hands, and then draw the finger up the other way to open the other side of the wrist.
8. Stay for a few minutes with a steady breath until you can feel the Qi intensify.
9. To come out release the arms and straighten out the legs and release.
10. Repeat on the other side.

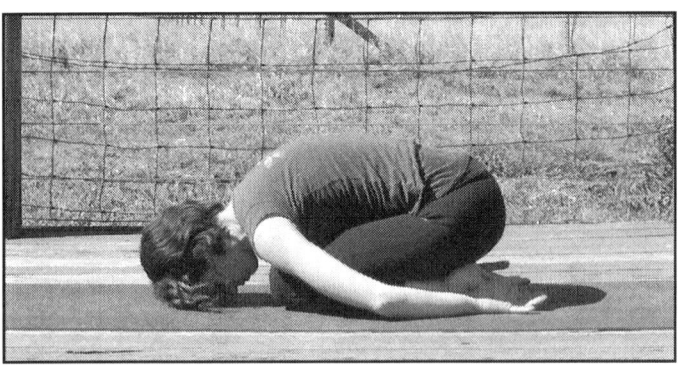

Child's Pose – Balasana

Main benefit – Calms the mind, cools the system, draws energy inside and softens the back.

1. Sit on your heels, feet flat in the seiza position. If it's too much on your ankles or knees, try placing a blanket under your feet and knees. If this doesn't work for you, then just come down into a cross-legged seated position.

2. From here, simply draw your torso down toward the floor. Rest your forehead on the floor. Relaxed arms can be out in front or down the side.

3. Close your eyes and take a few breaths, relax your back and shoulders.

4. When you're ready to come out, simply draw your torso back up to sit on your heels or on the floor.

- The child's pose can be done anytime you feel like you need to have a rest or break, especially in yoga class.

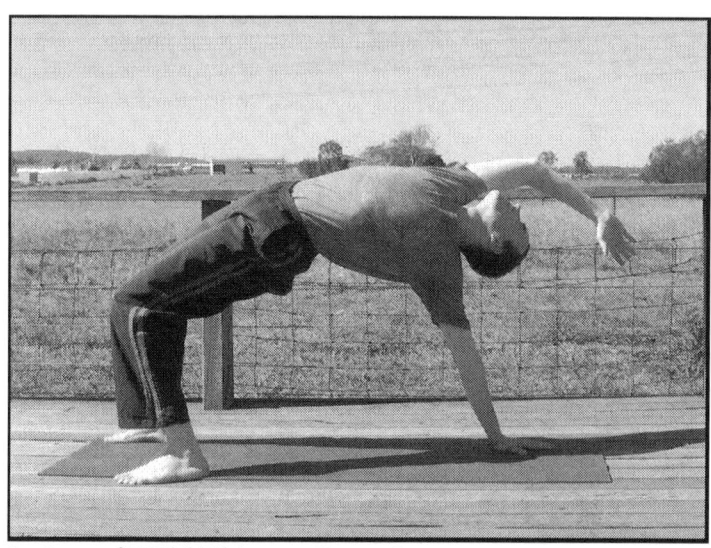

Variation of Wild Thing – Camatkarasana

Main Benefit – Opens the front of the torso, belly, lungs and chest.

Caution - This is an intermediate to advanced pose so only attempt it if you have been doing yoga for some time already.

1. Start in down facing dog.
2. Gently bend the knees and place your left foot underneath you and over the right side about 20cm or so to the side of your other foot.

3. Then keeping the knees bent slightly, allow the feet to pivot and draw the right arm off the floor to roll over into the backbend.
4. Extend the right arm behind you, and keep your hips working upwards.
5. Only hold for a breath or two and then to come out draw the right arm back in, pivot on the feet and then place the left foot back into the down facing dog position also placing the right hand back into down dog position.
6. Repeat to the other side.

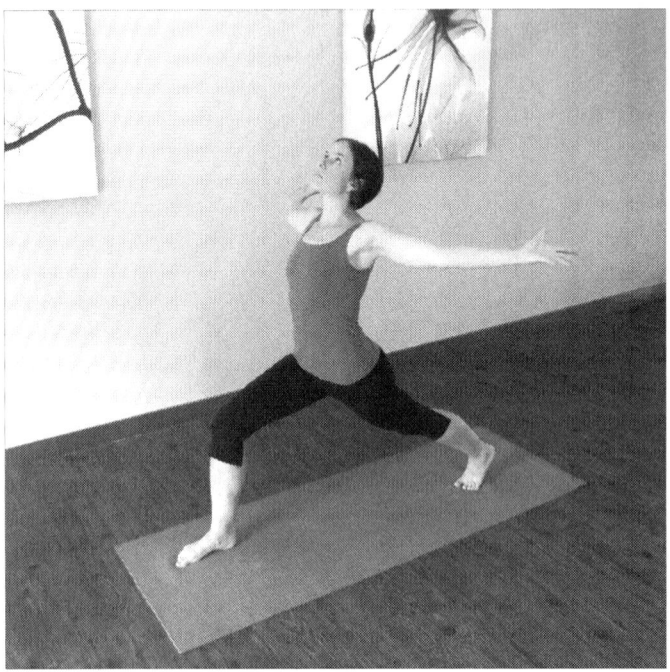

Warrior 1 Variation – Virabhadrasana 1
Main Benefit – Opens the heart and the channels on the arms while strengthening the legs.

1. Start by standing, with feet hip width apart at the front of your mat.

2. Bend the knees slightly to get balanced and step the left leg towards the back of the mat (about a leg length apart).
3. Bring the hands into prayer at the heart centre and allow the front knee to bend deeply. Let the back heel come off the mat as you try to keep the back leg long and straight.
4. When you feel settled, supported and strong in your legs open the arms up wide and gaze slightly up. Imagine giving the sky a big hug!
5. Allow your heart to open. Spread your fingers wide, keep your elbow and shoulder joints soft so the Qi can travel through them easily.
6. Hold for at least 3 deep and full breaths.
7. To come out, bring the hands back to heart centre and spring the back foot back up to the front of the mat.
8. Repeat on the other side.

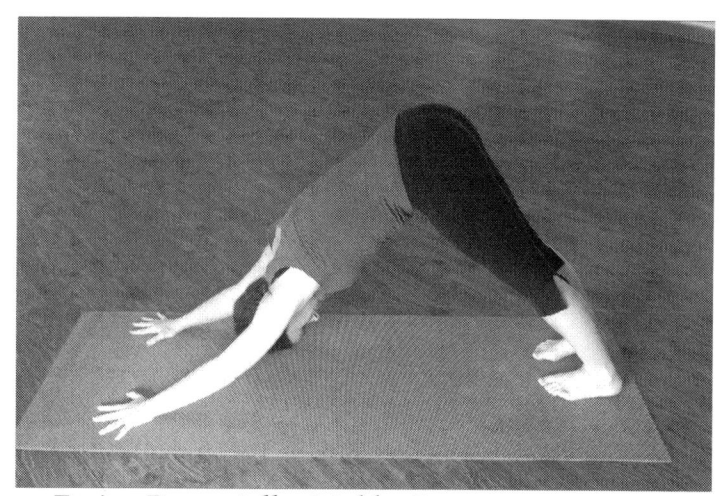

Down Facing Dog – Adho Mukha Svanasana

Main benefit – Strengthens and opens the arms, shoulders and legs.

1. Come onto all fours with hands underneath the shoulders and knees under the hips. Spread your fingers wide.

2. Tuck the toes under, start to extend the arms and start bringing the knees off the floor.
3. Come to extend the arms, and start to work the kegs straight. Try to bring the weight back into your legs and not so much into your arms.
4. Look to the floor just under your belly button.

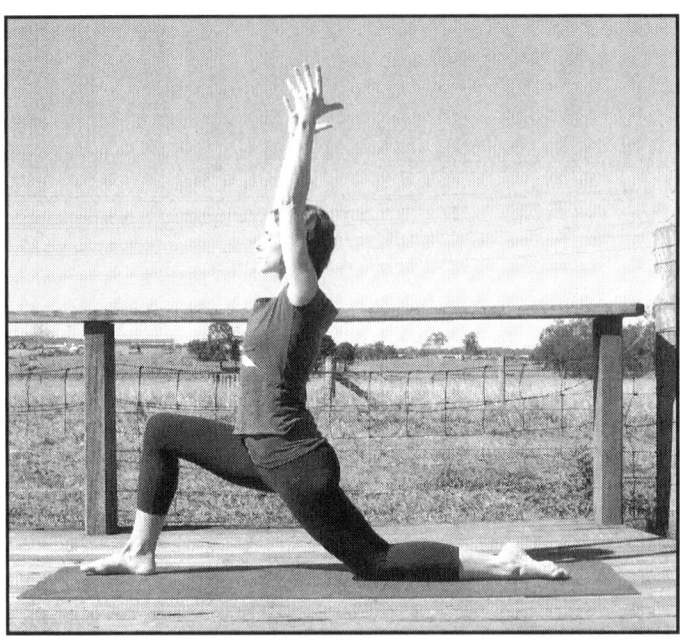

Low Lunge – Anjaneyasana
Main benefit – Opens the psoas muscle and opens the front of the body.

1. Ideally, you will start in a standing-forward, bent position (Uttanasana) at the front of the mat. Then simply step your left leg to the back of the mat and bring your back knee to the floor, the top of your back foot should be flat on the floor.
2. Make sure your front ankle is either just in front of or directly underneath your front knee.
3. Open your heart up and bring your arms out to the side, and then bring them up above your head. In this picture, the hands

are shoulder width apart – this makes it easier to relax the shoulders down away from the ears. You can bring your hands together too if that feels more natural.

4. Allow your lower back to lengthen and gently work your hips forward and down toward the floor, opening the front of your left hip.

5. After a few breaths, bring your torso and your arms down toward the floor, tuck your back toe under and step to the front of the mat, returning to your forward bend at the front of the mat.

6. Repeat on the other side.

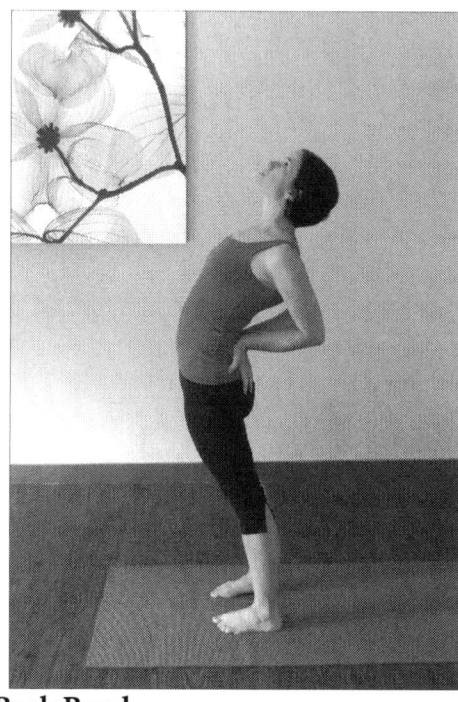

Standing Back Bend

Main Benefit – A back bend to strengthen the back of body and to open the heart.

1. Place your hands, onto the lower back with finger pointing downwards.

2. Draw the elbows towards each other, such the belly in before gently drifting the hips forward and leaning back.
3. Feel the heart and throat open. Only hold for a breath then come out.
4. Come out by drawing your torso forward and releasing the arms. Feel free to move the hips around in circles to release and then try again.

For more advanced practitioners, Camel Pose is recommended.

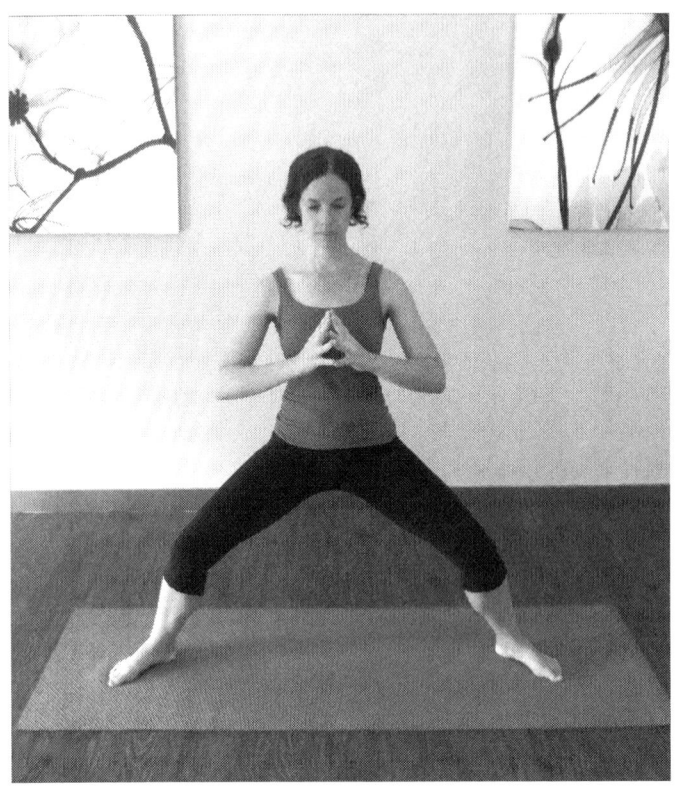

Horse Stance
Main benefit – Strengthens and grounds the legs into the earth and builds digestive fire.

1. Stand in the centre of your mat
2. Bring your legs wide apart (about 1 legs length apart)

3. Bring your hands into prayer position, relax the shoulders, arms are light.
4. Start to gently squat into your legs, keep the knees working back so your working the hips open.
5. Once you find a spot that you feel "switched on" and activated through the legs, hold it for some time.
6. Connect with your breath. Gently squeeze *Mula Bundha* (gentle squeeze of the anus muscle) and hold the posture.
7. Hold for at least 10 long steady breaths before slowly easing up and coming out of it.
8. Be sure to practice this a few times in each session. It's a great practice to do if you feel too "heady".

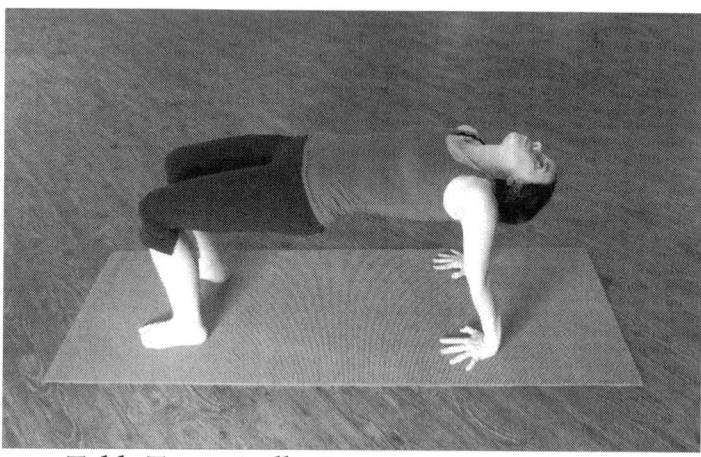

Reverse Table Top – Ardha Purvottanasana
Main Benefit – Strengthens the back of the body and opens the channels on the arms and on the front of the body.

1. Come to sit on your mat, with your knees bent and feet flat on the mat.
2. Bring your hands just behind you, fingers pointing forwards.
3. Start by raising the buttocks just off the floor.
4. If ok, raise the hips all the way so they are in line with your knees and shoulders.
5. Let your head rest back into the fold of the neck.

6. Get a sense of the shoulder working down away from the head. Allow the elbows to have a tiny bend in them, avoid hyperextending the elbow joint.
7. Plant your fingers and toes into the floor.
8. Connect with your breath and hold for around 5 long steady breaths.
9. To come out slowly lower your buttocks first, the head will naturally roll up without any effort.
10. Come to sit back on the mat.

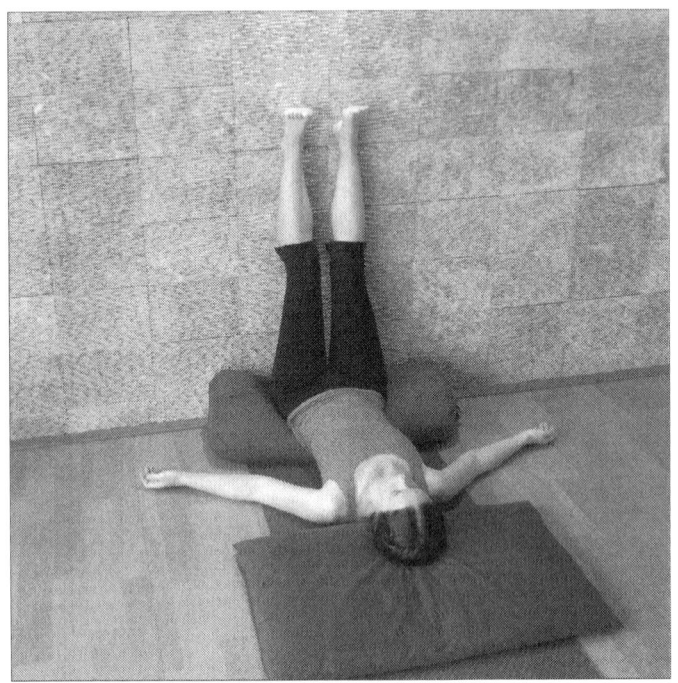

Legs Up the Wall – Viparita Karani
Main benefit – Drains the legs and nourishes the organs.

1. To get into this position can be a bit awkward. To start, the key is to sit up alongside the wall, as close as you can to the wall with one hip.
2. Then, you roll yourself down onto your back and shoot your legs up the wall. Ideally, your buttocks are quite close to the wall,

though for people who have tight hamstrings, they will need to come away from the wall so they can get their legs up, their knees will probably be bent, but that's ok. If your hamstrings are ok, wiggle yourself closer to the wall so your buttocks touch the wall.
3. Once you have found a comfortable position, let your arms fall away to the side, close your eyes and just relax with a gentle breath. You can stay here from anywhere between 3-15 minutes.
4. To come out, bend your knees, and then roll to your right side. Wait here for a minute or two so your legs can get some blood back into them before moving or standing. Take your time... if the phone rings or something like that, let it go... Do not rush out of this one.

Other techniques that regulate the Heart and Small Intestine:

Laughter Practice

Learning to laugh from deep within the belly is a profound and enjoyable experience. Laughing helps lengthen and stabilize the breath and naturally calms the mind and opens the mind/heart.

There are many yoga teachers who specialize in laughter practice and it is worth attending one of their classes to gain the full experience of laughing hysterically for extended periods of time with a bunch of other people.

You can practice it yourself of course. We have all experienced glimpses of it more often when we young. When you start laughing at something let yourself go. Let the laughter come from deep within your belly and allow your whole being to laugh. Eventually you will notice that you are not laughing at something that funny anymore, but you are simply laughing at laughing. The very act of laughing becomes joyful in itself.

Pranayama

Pranayama means breath control or regulation of prana (Qi). If you are pregnant, have high or low blood pressure, heat conditions or epilepsy please consult a health professional before embarking on pranayama techniques.

I would also advise not to practice pranayama too much (2+ hours each day) because it can be such a powerful practice that it can send people into mental instability due to its affect on the nervous system. If you interested in pranayama and want to practice it more seriously seek its important to find a verified and very experienced yoga teacher who can guide you properly into the world of pranayama.

Nadi Sodhana (one nostril breathing)

Main Benefit: Nadi Sodhana is a calming breath. It helps to regulate and balance the nervous system leaving the mind very clear and calm.

1. You can practice sitting up or lying down.
2. To start breathe out all the air from your lungs.
3. Using the thumb on your dominant hand, block your right nostril and breath in through the left nostril. Inhale the air into your belly and not just into your upper chest.
4. When you are 80% full of breath, seal off your left nostril with the ring finger of the same hand while keeping your right nostril closed and hold the breath for just one moment.
5. Then release the thumb on the right nostril and let the air exhale through the right nostril.
6. Once all the air is out start to inhale through that right nostril.
7. When you are 80% full, seal off your right nostril with your thumb again. Hold the breathe for one moment.
8. Then release the left nostril and let the air come out.

9. When the air is out, start to inhale through that left nostril.
10. Simply repeat this process, breathing in through one nostril, close, hold, release the air through the other nostril, then inhale through that nostril, close, hold and repeat for around 10 cycles.
11. When completed, relax your arm and body. Notice how you feel.

Hands to Heart

This practice simply involves place one or both hands over the chest and heart area and allowing the warmth of the hands to soften and relax the chest area. It is a very nurturing and calming practice you can do on yourself or on another person whenever it feels right.

Whenever you are anxious about a particular event that you are about to face it helps to simply stop for a moment just before you step into the room or wherever the event is to take place. Stop, place your hands on your heart, close down the eyes for a moment and then when you're ready, step forward into the room and into the unknown.

Hands into Prayer Position

Bringing the hands into prayer position balances out the nervous system and softens the heart. When you place your hands together the heart channels on both arms and hands connect up adding more support and energy to the heart and this is why there is a natural tendency to bring the palms together into prayer position when we wish to talk with or be humble in the presence of spirit.

You can add words of prayer, words of blessings or words of gratitude while hands are held in prayer position. It is also perfectly ok not to add any words to the practice. Bringing the hands together in prayer position and sensing the warmth in the palms can often be enough to sense a softening of the spirit.

Fire Element Daily Lifestyle Practices

- Stay up late dancing and having fun with friends

- Late to bed early to rise

- Set up inspirational meetings 11-1pm

- Seek out inspirational people and teachings

- Dream big. Write them down, share them with others and start putting them into action.

- Let go of being so serious, find more fun and joy.

- Avoid overthinking or over worrying because it can easily lead to anxiety and depression. To avoid falling into the pattern, get out more, attend a new yoga classes, meet up with friends, try something new.

- Connect with others, listen to their dreams and offer support if you can

- Don't do heavy thinking or decision making at night – save that for the day, let your nights be fun and creative.

- At from 7pm be sure to listen to your favorite music and get creative. Don't watch the news or read newspapers because at this time the heart energy is more susceptible and fragile – you want to nourish and nurture it at this time.

- Be open to new people and opportunities.

- Avoid too much time watching TV, reading or on a computer at night (over stimulation of the eyes disturbs the heart)

- Stay true to your path.

Supporting the Other Elements to Assist the Fire Element

As outlined in the 5-elements chapter, if we want to balance out the Fire element, we also need to take into consideration the elements that feed the Fire element which are Wood (*Shen* cycle) and Water (*Ko* cycle). This is especially the case of any illness or any disease related to the heart or small intestine, which often manifests as irregular body temperature, depression and mental instability.

Wood Element Stimulation and Harmonization

- Wood element likes to move so keep the body moving to avoid stagnation. Going for a walk can often be enough.
- Reduce or avoid alcohol, coffee, BBQ'd foods and smoking.
- De-clutter your environment, remove the non-essentials – spring clean
- Launch into new projects
- Get to bed before 11pm and wake early
- Lemon water on rising

Water Element Nourishment

- Keep cool. Cold showers and laying down to rest in the hottest part of the day can help to keep you cool
- Meditation, stillness and quiet time
- Good quality sleep
- Look after your kidneys with good quality water and keep hydrated
- Eat plenty of root vegetables

Food / Oriental Diet Therapy ~ Summer

For summer, the following foods and methods are recommended for nourishing and supporting the organs at this time of year:

Method of Cooking: Lightly cooked foods (steaming, poaching, stir-frying), small amounts of raw foods

Grains: Millet, barley, rye

Vegetables: Celery, spinach, cucumber, lettuce, greens, radish, asparagus, eggplants, cabbage, tomatoes, broccoli, cauliflower, zucchini, corn, beets, carrots, parsley, sprouts, watercress, bamboo shoots

Fruits: Apples, pears, watermelon

Beans and Nuts: Soy beans, mung beans, azuki beans, chick peas

Meat: Chicken, eggs, crab, tuna, oysters, and clams

Herbs and Seasonings (only if lacking fire): Black pepper, ginger, cinnamon, nutmeg, fennel

Avoid / Reduce
- Roasted, fried and deep fried foods
- Chilies
- Coffee and Chocolate
- Alcohol
- Vinegar

- Excess salt
- Cheese
- Ice-cream & ice water

Herbs to Support the Heart and Small Intestine

Here is a list of herbs that support the main organs involved in keeping the Heart and Small Intestine healthy.

Please seek guidance from a health professional (naturopath, herbalist, Chinese herbalist, Chinese medicine practitioner) for more information about correct dosages or for treating specific conditions.

Ginseng - Tones Qi and blood and supports the overall health and vitality of all organs

Ginko Biloba - Nourishes blood and increases blood flow to heart and brain

5-HTP - An amino acid (protein) that is very affective as an anti-depressant and helps people sleep

Acetyl L Carnetine - Invigorates mental function and works great as a natural energy motivator

Magnesium Citrate - Relaxes muscles throughout the body including the heart muscle. Helps to relax, sleep and recover.

Summer Meditations

Metta Meditation (Loving Kindness)

Preparation: Sit in a comfortable position. If you are sitting on the floor, I always recommend sitting up on a folded blanket – ideally, you want your knees to be just below your hips.

When you're in a comfortable seated position, place your hands in a comfortable position. I generally recommend interlacing your fingers and placing them on your lap or just in front of your lap, or simply place one palm on top of the other. When you place your hands this way, it generates a very nurturing energy and helps one draw the energy inward for regeneration. You can, of course, place your hands on your knees. This position, I find, tends to be more suited to an opening and expanding type of energy, good for sending out energy and metta (loving kindness).

Now, close your eyes and settle into a relaxed posture. Find your breath moving through your nostrils and keep watching it. Just keep your attention on your breath, let your mind's contents just move through without giving it much attention. Relinquish your mind's thoughts and images as they arise. Come back to your breath with an alert, yet relaxed awareness. Just watch your breath for at least five minutes until your mind starts to settle.

Now bring to mind
1. A picture of yourself. Visualize yourself happy, smiling, laughing and looking fully content. Hold the image and the feeling for about 1-2 minutes. (If you have difficulty with this then it is a sign of resistance, meaning that there is work to be

done and therefore returning to this Metta meditation practice in the near future would be worthwhile.)

2. Next bring a picture to your mind of someone who you deeply respect and admire. A person who represents profound love and understanding, like a highly evolved being or spiritual teacher for example. Picture them smiling with you, happy and fully in joy and love. Bathe in this image for about two minutes or so.

3. Next bring a picture to your mind of someone dearly beloved. Like a close family member or close friend. Picture them smiling, happy and content. Bathe in this image for about 1-2 minutes or so.

4. Next bring a picture to your mind of a neutral person. A person whom you have little or no strong feelings for, like the bus driver or a person that served you in the shop this morning. Picture them smiling, happy and content. Bathe in this image for about 1-2 minutes or so.

5. Next bring a picture to your mind of a hostile person. A person that you don't get along with, or a person who you regularly have arguments with, like a co-worker for example. Put your animosity aside and picture them smiling, happy and content. Bathe in this image for about 1-2mintues or so.

6. To finish bring the mind back to your breath and sense your body. Allow a little smile on your face as you send the loving kindness vibration you have cultivated to radiate and illuminate from your body. Imagine your body and heart like a light bulb that is sending out loving light in all directions. Bathe in this process for about 1-2 minutes or so.

When you are ready to come out, simply relax your posture and slowly open your eyes.

Mantra Meditation

Preparation: Sit in a comfortable position

When your mind has settled a little, move your awareness down to the centre of your chest, into the heart space
So as you breath in, focus your attention on this point and say to yourself, "Hummmmm", and as you breathe out, say to yourself, "Saaaaaaaa".
Do this for a few minutes.

Then move your attention to your third eye (between the eyebrows). We are working at connecting the heart with the energy of the mind so that the yin (heart) and yang (mind) can balance out and work together. As you inhale, focus your attention the third eye and say to yourself, "Hummmmm", and as you exhale, say to yourself, "Saaaaaaaa".

Do this for a few minutes.

After a few minutes, let go of the practice. Let yourself simply sit for a moment or two.

Then allow a gentle smile to come onto your face, an effortless smile. Then begin to visualize that gentle smile moving down to your heart space area. Give thanks to your heart by smiling gently at it and let the smile radiate out into the entire chest area.

To complete this meditation, bring your attention back to your breath at your nostrils. Let go of all other practices. Watch your breath until you feel calm and relaxed. Then when ready, open your eyes gently and release your posture.

Conclusion

You would have already realized by now that Oriental yoga is not just a yoga system full of postures, but is actually a complete system for living. As we become more aware of the natural laws of life and how they influence us inside and out, it becomes a very humbling experience. We learn that these natural forces are so powerful that we can do little but simply yield to their strength and beauty but this yielding doesn't act to take our energy away but actually reinforces our inner strength and power. When we learn to yield in this way, the ego and mind naturally becomes quiet, and only then can the true self rise up from within and shine forth. The doorway to the heart is then opened and once that door is open, keep walking on the path and don't turn back. May the force be with you!

~ May All Beings Be Happy ~

Recommended Reading

Ted Kaptchuk, *The Web That has No Weaver: Understanding Chinese Medicine* (Rosetta Books, 2010)

Harriet Beinfield, Afram Korn, *Between Heaven and Earth: A Guide to Chinese Medicine* (Ballantine Books, 1992)

B.K.S. Iyengar, *Light on Yoga: Yoga Dipika* (Schocken, Revised Edition 1995)

Martin Kirk, Brooke Book, Daniel DiTuro, *Hatha Yoga Illustrated* (Human Kinetics, 2005)

Suzanne Friedman, *Heal Yourself with Qi Gong* (New Harbinger Publications, 2009)

Lao Tzu, Stephen Mitchell, *Tao Te Ching: An Illustrated Journey* (Frances Lincoln, 2009)

Resources

Yoga Supplies (mats, bolsters, blankets, etc)

USA
www.manduka.com

www.gaiam.com

www.barefootyoga.com

UK
www.yogamatters.com

www.yogamad.com

Australia
www.iyogaprops.com.au

www.empind.com.au

Yoga Music

www.soundstrue.com

Other Books By This Author

www.michaelhetherington.com.au

Chakra Balancing Made Simple and Easy

How to Do Restorative Yoga

Autumn Oriental Yoga

Meditation Made Simple

The Little Book of Yin

How to Learn Acupuncture

Printed in Great Britain
by Amazon